MARY LLEWELLYN

A Cat Has Nine Lives

And So Do You

Nine Steps to Health and Wellness

D1740820

By

Alister Bredee

Alister Bredee

Publishing History

BSC E-Publishing

www.billsmart.com/bsc/e-publishing

Paperback Edition 1 / January 2017
ISBN-13: 978-1540819260
ISBN-10: 978-1540819264

Dedication

This book is dedicated to all those people who have put their trust in me and my methods over the years. I particularly salute Dr. Harry Howell for being my mentor and teacher. Thank- you Harry for opening the box.

Acknowledgements

This all came about when I came to Koh Samui in 2007 and started to work in the "detox" industry. This book is a culmination of that work. Thank-you Graham Rowe for giving me working space at Health Oasis. Thank-you Claire Bostock for having enough faith to bring me to Absolute Sanctuary. Thank-you Tom for helping make Health Ambit Consultancy a reality. Thank-you Dr. Tara for helping to get all of this off the ground. Thank-you Pummaret Sangtong for being my partner through thick and thin. Meister Eckhart tells us there is only one prayer which is..."Thank-you God."

Table of Contents

Table of Figures

Preamble

"No Disease Can exist inside a clean body."

Dr. Edward Group

"Let Food be Thy Medicine."

Hippocrates

"Negative thoughts can kill you faster than a bad germ. We have to detoxify the mind."

Dr. Antonio Jimenez

"When Growth stops decay sets in."

Dr. Rashid Buttar

"Detox Reduces Your Toxic Exposure."

Dr. Veronique Desaulniers

Foreword

I was waiting to see the Consultant. He swaggered into the ward, sporting a brushed brown Armani suit. Turning to me he said; "We'll put you on 6 months chemotherapy treatment," and briskly moved on. He was halted by a middle-aged woman, who asked, "what about the side effects of chemotherapy?" Smiling, he answered patronizingly whilst patting her on the shoulder, "there, there, let us worry about those details", and he hastened on.

As a practitioner of Holistic Medicine with 8 years of clinical practice under my belt at the time; I was astounded! As I glanced around that oncology ward, I wondered how many of those patients would still be around in five years' time. That was in 1999.

In that instant, I made a decision to become and remain a cancer survivor without recourse to chemotherapy.

It has taken me 17 years to come out with that story. I am still here. I see myself as a "whole-life healer". I overcame that challenge and against the odds. I have dedicated my life to health and healing. If I can do it so can you.

This book is not a novel. It is a self-help guide devoted to your wellness. Please allow me to show you the path." Alister Bredee D.HH, D.CN

Introduction

Welcome to "A Cat Has Nine Lives And So Do You 9 Steps To Health and Wellness". This is a journey, and the journey is all about you. How you take this journey is up to you. But here is our mission statement:

"If you can effectively detoxify the body, cancer, heart disease and neurotoxicity cannot exist."

That's a pretty big statement, isn't it? In short by effective detoxification, 92% of all diseases cannot exist. Cancer and Heart Disease are on the increase. The bottom line is we are individually responsible for our own health. It's not your Dr. it's not your Consultant, it's not your Naturopath it's you. Are you willing to step up and take ownership of the responsibility? If you are ill, it is not because you are pharmaceutically disadvantaged; the reason is that some underlying root cause lurks under the symptoms and it needs addressing. Don't treat the symptoms find and heal the cause. I liken this to removing the bulb when the oil pressure warning light glows red whilst driving. The annoying red light goes out (the symptom) but the cause has not been addressed, which means the engine is in great danger of seizing up (the cause). Tracking the cause and acting on it, is likely to save you a stack of cash in repair bills. Isn't that the most sensible route to take?

This journey is designed to wake you up and make you aware; awake to your own health and some of the steps you can take to preserve this precious gift. Many take health for granted and only get concerned when something goes wrong. Once a problem arises we rush off to a health care professional to have the matter sorted. Isn't it better to make good health an ongoing target? Wellness becomes the intention and not illness. You can do that yourself. Yes, we sometimes need guidance and assistance and that is what "A Cat Has Nine Lives And So Do You "is all about. The book is designed to help you achieve wellness on a consistent basis. Are you up for it? OK, then step up to the marker and make this pledge to yourself.

"I am responsible for my own health and I am willing to take on that responsibility."

I appreciate the weight of that responsibility. Well, done for taking it on. That is, indeed, something to boast about. Give yourself a well-deserved pat on the back and follow it up with a happy dance. The content, here, might be serious but let's have some fun working it!

Don't wait for illness to show-up. Once *"dis-ease"* has somatized into the body, it's too late! It is in the physical and that makes healing difficult. Let's instead, take charge and work to rid ourselves of the poisons and toxins that have given rise to the "*dis-ease*" state in the first place. Doesn't that make sense?

I truly understand that this takes time, effort and commitment, but you are not alone on this momentous voyage. But we at Health Ambit Consultancy are here to guide and help you through "A Cat Has Nine Lives And So Do You *" in an effort* that your immune system performs optimally and that keeps sickness at bay. The choice is yours of course, but you are not on your own, we, too, are dedicated to your success. All you have to do is reach out and we are there for you. I suspect that makes this "*Program*" unique.

There are 9 Steps in "A Cat Has Nine Lives And So Do You." You can complete it all in a relatively short time space; the pace is really up to you. It is important you feel comfortable with each step and the changes that occur in your health. You can have negative reactions as you begin to shed the toxins of mind, body and spirit. Be re-assured, they pass, usually quite quickly, perhaps in no more than a day or two. However, when you are complete, you will find that you have made some significant life altering changes. Are you ready to begin?

The 9 Steps are:

There are 10 really, as we begin with *the Basics* but we don't include these in the total as they provide a starting place for everybody. These are changes you need to make in order to get on board with the *Program*. *The Basics* are arguably the area in which, if you like most of the people on the planet, will need to make the most alteration. Some people, on the other hand, will have already embraced many of these health-enhancing tools and that is fantastic and some will have a little work to do; that too is fantastic.

Life 1: The Kidney Cleanse. Before we start cleansing the gut we need to start with the urinary system as this supports the digestive system. Pesticides and heavy metals abound and we need to eradicate them from the body.

Life 2: The Mother of all Organs is the Gut. Most diseases start in the digestive tract. It's really important to detoxify the colon, the small intestine and the stomach. How do we do this? We clean up the diet and cleanse the colon with colonics, enemas or our own proprietary herbal detox formula.

Life 3: The Power of a Liver Cleanse. The liver is the largest organ; it acts as the chemical factory. Although it cleanses toxins, it accumulates them, too. This interferes with the digestive process and backs–up to hinder the immune system.

Life 4: Cleaning the Lymphatic System. The lymphatic system is a network of tissues and organs that help get rid of toxins. The primary function of lymphatic fluid, made up of white blood cells, is to fight infection. The lymphatic system is similar to the circulatory system, only larger and it does not possess a pump. That means it can get blocked easily. We need ways to clear it, so it functions efficiently.

Life 5: The Parasite Cleanse. Most people have worms! It's is relatively easy to kill the parasites, but steering clear of infection induced by the eggs and the larvae is another story. We can be infected by our pets, poor bathroom habits, our finger nails and even door knobs. Dr. Hulda Clark believed parasites lay behind all major illnesses. It's no good embarking on a five-minute clean-up. This is a much longer tale which has been largely ignored by Western Medicine.

Life 6: Cleansing Heavy Metals. Heavy Metals like mercury, lead, cadmium, aluminum and arsenic abound on this industrially polluted planet. Mercury is considered to be the most toxic substance on Earth following the radioactive elements like plutonium, yet it is found in fish, is used in dentistry and the preservative Thimerosal is accepted as an anti-fungal and antiseptic agent; used in vaccines. Some claim it plays a substantial part in the current autism epidemic. These metals accumulate in organs and we need a method of chelating or getting rid of them.

Life 7: The Emotional Detox. This is arguably the most important in "A Cat Has Nine Lives And So Do You." Toxic emotions block the body's energy pathways. These trapped emotions create symptoms that can be much more life threatening than any bacteria or virus. This "detox" helps you release the emotions. All negative emotions are related to the Chinese Meridian System. Once they have been removed we show you a simple and user-friendly method you can use yourself to clear issues as they arise.

Life 8: The Dangers of Electrical Stress. Today we are surrounded by EMFs (low level electrical magnetic fields). They come to us through our current obsession with EMF technology in the form of mobile phones, microwave ovens and computers. They are the source and the unseen electromagnetic waves that surround us every day of our lives. In this "detox" we examine the often unreported dangers posed by this new energy form and look at ways to protect ourselves from what can only be described as "dirty electricity".

Life 9: The Spiritual Cleanse. This is a hugely important topic, comprising an area that many are blissfully unaware. We encourage you to step outside the realm of self with its self-centered certainty that we are all different. No, we are not, we are all "one" when everything is reduced to the bare essentials. The "Course in Miracles" informs us there are only two emotions, love and fear and everything else is a variant on the same theme. In my point of view, it's simpler than that. There are only two emotions, one feels heavy, dark, restricted, uncomfortable and draining, whilst the other feels light, bright, airy, breezy, open and easy. Which one of these would you choose? This "detox" shows you how to make the "light" choice.

Those then are the 9 Lives. Now, what?

Congratulations you bought the book, in whichever format it came in. What are you going to do with it?

Mission Statement

"Our job is to inspire others to recognize that different possibilities exist, are credible, and different realities can be created by living those possibilities which create a different reality."

How does it Work?

You can use *"A Cat Has Nine Lives And So Do You"* as a self-help guide and let it inform and assist you make some important changes in your life.

If you feel *"a do-it-yourself"* approach is overwhelming, then you can sign-up for a guided program. This means I act as your mentor and help, encourage and support you through the program. Your *"9 steps"* becomes interactive for you. This is how it works.

Silver Package: A one-off sign-up fee entitles you to 4X45 minute Skype/or person to person sessions with me as well as reasonable e-mail contact. During our meetings, I will answer all your questions and coach you through the *"detox"* as well as keep you on track. This practically guarantees that you commit to the Program and grasp the intended results. If you genuinely want to take charge of your health and well-being, this is the recommended route.

Gold Package: This is the even more committed approach and the one-off sign-up fee entitles you to 8X45 minutes Skype or person to person appointments with me as well as weekly e-mail contact and the provision of an extra emergency session if need be. During the meetings, I will personally help you through each of the *"9 steps"*. This will give you the knowledge and skill to proceed confidently to the end of the Program, so achieving the health benefits you so earnestly seek. This is only for the truly committed.

Platinum De-Luxe: The content is the same as *"The Gold Package"*. However, this one includes the bonus of *"Home Detox Kit"*. The "Kit" comprises a prime collection of cleansing herbs for you to turn into delicious shakes which enable you to complete your own cleansing at home for 8 days. You don't need intrusive enemas or colonics but to make this experience even more effective they would add an advantage. This Program is professionally designed offering a natural herbal cleansing, supported by a healthy eating regime. It is intended to detox the body at a deep cellular level whilst producing moderate weight loss as an additional bonus. This is, indeed, the definitive choice for somebody truly dedicated to making giant strides to enhance their health, wellness and longevity.

"Homestay Program: ", can be compressed into an 8 or 10 day stay on the delightful tropical island of Koh Samui. You get here and we fix you up with suitable accommodation. You enjoy the *"shakes"* that are freshly prepared for you several times per day as well as a healthy living foods meal. You have the opportunity to attend regular yoga classes, walk on the beach and swim in the sea, enjoy massages that are fine tuned for you. Our colonic therapist is a true healer, who uses the treatments not only to clean the *"mother of all organs"* but to diagnose conditions that can be addressed during your stay on Samui and beyond. The Kidney Cleanse and the Basics commence before you leave home. The Gut, the Liver, the Lymphatic, the Emotional and Spiritual *"detox"* all take place during your visit to Samui. We start you off on the Parasite, Lymphatic, Heavy Metal and Electrical Stress components here in Thailand but you will need to continue the work when you return home. Have no fear we do not simply abandon you but continue with coaching and counseling once you get back home. For full details of *"The Homestay"*, please contact us at Health Ambit Consultancy.

healthambitconsultancy@protonmail.com

As a point of fact, if any of the packages catch your eye, please contact us by e-mail and we can then schedule a cost free time to talk to you directly by Skype, What's App or Line when we can answer your queries directly and clarify anything that seems unclear, help you select the Program that is most suitable for you and then bring you aboard for something that is sure to change your life.

To schedule a conversation with us, e-mail.

healthambitconsultancy@protonmail.com

The Crux of the Matter......Inflammation

Inflammation is a term that is much bandied about but what does it mean? OK let's start at the beginning. The principal reason for *"detoxing"* is to substantially reduce poisons in the system. *"Detoxing"* reduces inflammation because it destroys FREE RADICALS. To grasp what these little rascals are about we need to examine, atoms, the building blocks of our Universe. Atoms consist of a nucleus, neutrons, protons and electrons. The number of protons (positively charged particles) contained in the atom's nucleus determines the number of electrons (negatively charged particles) surrounding the atom. An Oxygen atom has 8 protons; that means there are 2 electrons in the inner shell and 6 in the outer which adds up to the necessary 8. Electrons are very important because they are required for chemical reactions to take place, and go on to form molecules, which are the next biggest structures after atoms.

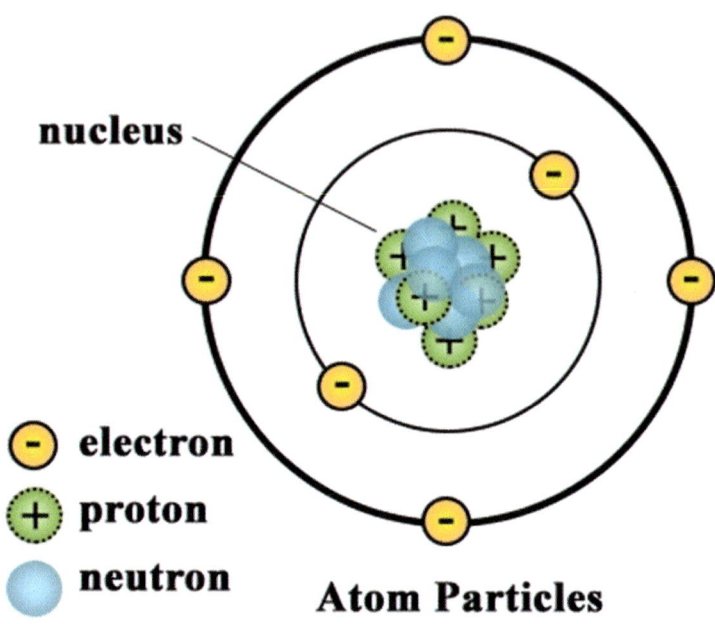

Atom Particles

© Buzzle.com
Figure 1

Generally speaking, the bonds do not split, because that would leave an unpaired electron out in the cold. But sometimes bonds are weak, whilst toxins make them even weaker. When these weakened bonds split all hell is let loose as free radicals are created. A free radical is a crazed unpaired electron rushing off to link up with another. This makes the whole structure extremely unstable. Stability can only return when the single electron finds a mate and becomes a couple once again. This chain reaction wages war in a living cell and like a bush fire soon spreads to other cells. The human body comprises trillions of cells; free radical devastation soon leaps to other cells, destabilizing cell after cell. When metal is exposed to water it rusts. Free radicals act similarly. Like rusted metal the process is weakening, so cells break down completely. The cell membrane is damaged which in turn destroys the lipids that live within the cell itself. The name for this is lipid peroxidation. The powerful oxidative explosion lasts for no more than a Nano-second. The ensuing damage is called inflammation, and the inflammatory response arising from the split second oxidative reaction can persist hours after the actual event. What creates these toxins that give rise to the free-radicals? The worst offenders are heavy metals namely lead, cadmium, mercury, arsenic and aluminum. Another enemy on this particular battle-field comprises "POPs". These translate as "Persistent Organic Pollutants"; such baddies don't biodegrade. Meaning they tend to hang around in the atmosphere for a long time. They come in the form of pesticides, pharmaceuticals and other pollutants. DDT was banned many years ago but provides a classic example of a *"POP"*. Chemicals like this leach into the soil; when crops are grown, the poisons have a means of entering the food chain. When we eat the produce, the result is inflammation!

Smoking, for example, exposes the smoker to substantial free-radical damage. This causes cellular injury as well as oxidative stress. Yes, we can off-set free radical damage by using anti-oxidants like Vitamins, A, C and E. They work because they produce the missing electrons that the crazed free-radicals are smashing through cells to find. Taking anti-oxidants is hugely important just as eating anti-oxidant rich foods like fresh fruit and vegetables. Yes, both measures reduce inflammation, but we need to go one step further. That means it's essential we change destructive habits and make better lifestyle choices. To make this worthwhile it is also critical to remove the toxic free-radical inducers from our lives and from our bodies. The paramount way to reach this target is to *"De-Toxify"*. And that my friends are what "A Cat Has Nine Lives And So Do You *"is* all about.

If you suffer from an inflammatory *"dis –ease"* like asthma, peptic ulcers, rheumatoid arthritis, periodontitis, ulcerative colitis, Crohn's Disease, sinusitis or much, much more, this *"de-tox"* is essential for you. If you go to your Dr. with an inflammatory condition, more than likely he or she will prescribe a NSAID or a non-steroid anti-inflammatory drug. The idea is these medicines stop prostaglandins which are lipid based, hormone-like substances. For instance, aspirin is a NSAID. Prostaglandins supposedly suppress the condition, but actually they contribute to inflammation, pain and fever. The question is are these drugs the real answer? The response is *"no"* because such treatments address the symptoms and not the cause of the problem. Besides many NSAIDs have serious side-effects which include heart attacks and strokes. Fever, by the way, is good, not bad, contrary to popular understanding. Providing fever is controlled, it demonstrates the immune system is working optimally and is actually fighting *"dis-ease"*. This increased activity causes the rise in body temperature. When you suppress the temperature with a NSAID like aspirin or paracetamol the fever reduces but so does the immune response.

Of course, it would be foolish to stamp out all free-radical activity. If something exists it has a purpose. What we seek, however, is a balance. Lack is dangerous, an excess is hazardous but balance equates to good health and harmony. That's where we all want to be.

The Basics

To move towards health and well-being many of us will have to make some changes. Of course, the fewer changes the better. If most of what follows does not apply to you, well done! Chances are you are a lot closer to your "Health and Fitness" objectives than many other people.

Our objective is to reduce inflammation as far as possible.

Diet and Exercise

Regarding diet, the objective is to eat healthily. What does that mean? The most important item to regulate is sugar. In a nutshell, it is important to grasp that sugar impairs the immune system. Higher blood sugar readings harm phagocyte activity. Phagocytes are immune cells whose job is to protect the body by gobbling up harmful foreign particles like bacteria and dead cells. Their presence is essential in fighting infection and creating immunity. The most effective phagocytes include several types of white blood cells; they include neutrophils, monocytes and macrophages. Anti-aging expert Dr. Norman Shealy explains:

"There are four essential habits: no smoking, body mass index of between 18 to 25, eating five or more servings

combined of fruits and vegetables a day (I say a minimum of 7), exercising the minimum of thirty minutes five days a week (I say 35). Three percent of Americans do all of those. We still have 22% smoking, 7% of people overweight, with 33% of those obese. The average American consumes 2.2 servings of fruits and vegetables and only 10% of people get that minimum amount of exercise. If all Americans suddenly develop those four habits, within twenty years, life expectancy in the United States will go from an average of 78 years to one hundred."

My comment: THIS DOES NOT ONLY APPLY TO THE USA. The UK life-expectancy figure is higher at 81.5 and Japan higher still at 83. Thailand ties with Sri Lanka at 74.9. To achieve these numbers, regular exercise is essential. Choose something you like and stick to it. You need to spend the minimum of 35 minutes per day at it. Walking will do, but you need to walk briskly so you get out of breath and raise your heart rate. Walking up a hill is much better than on the flat. Moving the body helps circulate blood and lymph fluid. The greater the circulation the more the liver can do its job of detoxification. Running, brisk walking, bicycling, dancing and swimming are all excellent examples. Aerobics, Hatha yoga, Pilates and the martial arts encourage stretching, suppleness and overall aerobic wellness. Take your pick of one or more of these and practice for the minimum of 35 minutes at least 5 times per week. *"The Five Tibetan Rites"* is a system of yoga based exercises that most can do at home. This systemic exercise ritual is said to be more than 2500 years old. The exercises were first publicized by Peter Kelder in an interesting book entitled *"Eye of Revelation"* published in the USA in 1939.

You might prefer to see how the exercises are done on YouTube. These videos show 21 repetitions of each of the exercises. However, depending on your state of fitness begin slowly, starting with 3 repeats of each of the exercises and then gently increase until you reach 21 which is the maximum permitted in a single session. The breathing is important so watch the video carefully.

https://www.youtube.com/watch?V=nCRY8AUJxVW

Sugar

A study was published in the August 2000 issue of *"The Journal of Clinical Endocrinology and Metabolism"* that came from the University of Buffalo in Upper New York State. The study team was led by Dr. Paresh Dandora, who happened to be a Professor of Medicine at the University. Their findings showed how excess sugar stimulates the formation of free-radicals. The resulting inflammation from sugar ingestion initiated the formation of plaque which is dangerous because it blocks arteries. Late Onset Diabetes (Type 2) is also linked to free-radical generation. Dandora and his team of scientists gave 14 healthy people who had fasted for 12 hours, 75 grams of glucose dissolved in 300 mg of water. This is about the equivalent in sugar content of two cans of Coca-Cola. The control group of 6 drank a water saccharine solution instead. This type of test is called a Blood Sugar Tolerance Test. They are extremely revealing. Blood samples were taken at the fasting level and then one, two and three hours afterwards. The blood samples revealed that the control group who drank saccharine water showed no changes over the 3 hour test period. The glucose group had dramatically different results; their samples divulged free-radical generation had increased significantly after one hour and more than doubled after two. At the same time levels of Vitamin E, a powerful anti-oxidant fell by 4% at hour 2 and were still substantially depleted at hour 3. To decrease inflammation; the key to all *"dis-ease"*, it's essential we stop eating sugar. It is easily as addictive as cocaine and it alters brain chemistry. Another Research Team, this time from the Princeton Neuroscience Institute, illustrated that rats eating large quantities of sugar when hungry underwent neurochemical brain changes that were very similar to those produced by drugs like cocaine, morphine and nicotine. The team concluded that *"sugar-bingeing"* causes long- lasting effects that increase the inclination to take other drugs, particularly ALCOHOL. In 1931 Dr. Otto Warburg won the Nobel Prize in Physiology for his discovery that cancer cells are metabolically limited to feed on sugar. Sugar has no place in a health conscious lifestyle. Those empty calories cause obesity, vitamin and mineral loss and of course inflammation through free-radical damage.

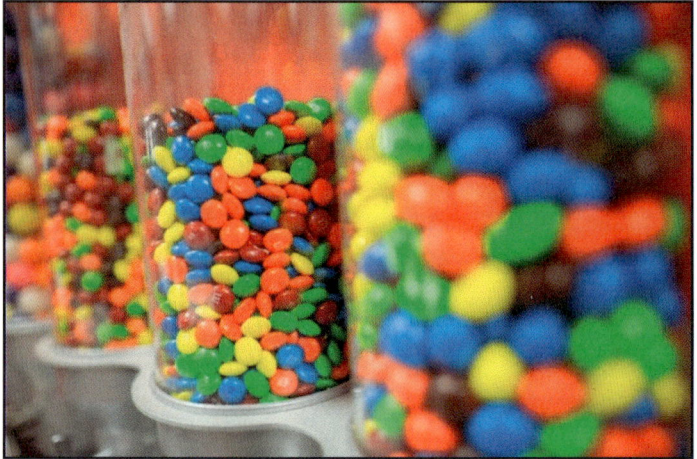

Figure 2

How to Stop Sugar
- Stop adding sugar to food or drinks.
- Stop buying sugar laden processed foods.
- Stop eating milk chocolate (dark chocolate with 85% cacao is OK)
- Stop munching on sweets, biscuits and sugary desserts.
- Stop those soft drinks that come in cans.
- Stop buying fruit juices in cartons. They are full of sugar. Make your own.

Is this a tall order or a worthwhile challenge?

You will be surprised, as you reduce sugar consumption the desire for sweet and sugary foods begins to wane. If you feel in need of help. E-mail us at:

Healthambitconsultancy@protonmail.com

And we'll assist you!

Interestingly, Dr. Dandora's study found that eliminating sugar fostered weight loss. Moreover, when over-weight people lost weight there was a commensurate reduction in free-radicals. Now, there's a way to go! Oh, if you need a healthy sweetener, try Stevia. Unlike other artificial sweeteners this one is plant based coming from a South American species; part of the Asteraceae family that is related to the daisy. Stevia is 200 times sweeter than sugar, has 0 calories whilst containing minerals including iron. It does not spike blood sugar so it can safely be ingested by those with a blood sugar issue. All in all, this is a hugely better option than sugar. Try it if you have a sweet tooth!

Grains

Americans are urged to eat 6-11 servings of grain products daily, including at least 3 servings of fiber-rich whole grains. The Authorities are allowing some of these products to carry health benefit claims, proclaiming they reduce cancer and heart disease. Many nutritionists and experts vehemently disagree with this notion. Dr. Loren Cordain a Professor at Colorado State University is one of them. He draws from a little-known book edited by Dr. A.P Simopoulos entitled, *"Cereal Grains. Humanity's Double Edged Sword"*. Seventeen plant species provide 90% of the world's food supply, without these plants it would be impossible to feed the 7.3 billion souls who inhabit Earth. It seems that approximately 15000 years ago fossil records demonstrate that large animal populations started to decline. This put an end to the hunter-gatherer lifestyle that was then in existence. In that time archaeologists found evidence of settlements and remains of crude ground stones and mortars. The age of agriculture had dawned. People stopped their dependence on wild meat, fruit, vegetables and nuts and started to eat a grain based diet which was completely incompatible with their previous ways. In order to grow crops the nomadic way had to stop and the population began to form settlements. Shortly afterwards interesting facts started to reveal themselves. Skeletal remains showed body size decreased and there was also evidence of diseases that would be compatible with a more sedentary way of being. These included cardiovascular disease, cancer, diabetes, high blood pressure as well as bone disease. These settlements have made possible the way of life we know today. As the villages grew into communities hostilities occurred with neighbors; so evolved the concept of war. In the Western World 50% of the caloric intake comes from bread, whilst in Asia, South America and Africa cereal crops comprise 80% of the diet. What then is wrong with grains? For the most part nothing; true they don't contain much vitamin C and only tiny traces of B12. Vitamin B12 deficiency (frequently lacking in vegetarians) causes megaloblastic anemia which can be the basis of cognitive difficulties as well as vascular disease. However, one thing is strikingly clear...wheat, barley, rye and oats as well as durum, spelt and kamut contain gluten. Gluten is as its name suggests, a type of glue. It is a mixture of proteins that keep the food together and helps dough rise. Bread has a high gluten content, whilst the leaching and kneading of pastry reduce, often with water, the gluten content. Gluten triggers inflammation. It can damage the intestines resulting in leaky gut syndrome; overall it is best avoided not only by celiacs but by all of us. Here is the test: eliminate all grains from your diet for a period of two weeks. At the end of the two weeks check how you feel. Do you feel lighter, brighter more energized and breezy? Then it is best for you to avoid grains entirely. If you don't notice much difference, start to re-introduce gluten once again. If you see the change, stop! If nothing happens, you are OK with grains and can consume them freely.

Start Taking Anti-Oxidants

Anti-oxidants help eradicate free radical damage. These compounds offer up electrons so that free-radicals can be paired off. This stops the rampage of damage resulting inflammation. Vitamin C (ascorbic acid) is as cheap as chips. Buy the crystalline form and add the powder to smoothies and juices. One small teaspoon is roughly 5 Grams. That's the place to start. If you take too much you are likely to get loose stools. Realize this is one of the ways toxins are eliminated. It is inconvenient, though. If this occurs cut back the dose, simply put less powder on the spoon and the symptoms will disappear. If you choose the tablet form, select 1 gram pills that contain bio-flavonoids, which make the vitamin more effective. Linus Pauling, the father of mega-dose vitamin therapy, recommended a minimum daily dose of 2000 mg of Vitamin C.

The Dangers of Trans Fatty Acids

These are unsaturated fats that do not occur in nature. That means they are man-made. The most common example is margarine. Margarine was feverishly marketed as a safer alternative to saturated fats like butter. This advertising frenzy largely dreamed up by copywriters erroneously, proclaimed, the margarines to be heart healthy and butter dangerous because it contained cholesterol. Trans Fats are industrial products made from vegetable oils that are heated. Incidentally heating a polyunsaturated oil does not create TFAs contrary to popular opinion. But re-using the cooking oil many times does; the same applies to healthful olive oil. DO NOT RE-USE COOKING OIL. The problem with Trans Fatty Acids is they are hydrogenated.

Hydrogen is added to the liquid oils to make them more solid. Effectively this changes them to polymers. These long chain molecules are similar to rubber or plastics. The supposed Fats go to make margarine and purportedly "heart healthy" spreads as a replacement for butter. 1) **Please stop using these products**. 2) TFAs are cheap to produce, easy to use and have a long shelf-life, so they are a popular choice for inclusion in packaged or processed foods. They are marked on labels as *"partially hydrogenated oils"*. These oils are not safe because they create substantial free-radical damage, which as you now know contributes to inflammatory conditions like for example atherosclerosis, a major cause of heart disease. 3) **STOP BUYING PROCESSED FOODS.** Trans Fats are found in foods like doughnuts (full of sugar too) frozen pizza, cakes and biscuits. If you buy these foods, be sure to look at labels very carefully. Many restaurants, particularly the fast food variety, use Trans Fats to deep fry. They use the oils many times in their deep fryers. My Professor Dr. Harry Howell claimed that these restaurants sold the old oil to processors who then refined, bleached and then re-processed it to make margarine. 4) **STOP EATING IN FAST FOOD RESTAURANTS.** Instead eat lots of healthy fats like butter, olive and coconut oil. Do not re-use cooking oils and be sure to add lots of anti-oxidant rich fruit and vegetables to your diet.

Eat the Rainbow

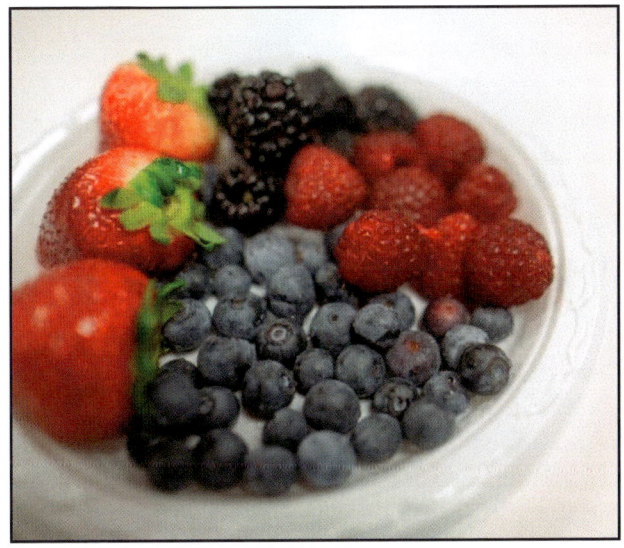

Figure 3

Be sure to include at least 7 servings of fruit and vegetables to your diet daily. 7 servings are the minimal but 10 would be optimal. But beware..."*POPs*" or Persistent Organic Pollutants which come by way of fertilizers and pesticides that are liberally sprayed onto the crops by the growers to enhance their productivity and profit. You can't blame the producers; they want to make a living just like anybody else. However, it is your responsibility **to thoroughly wash your fruit and veggies.** Yes, the Supermarket might have done so, but you need to make sure! Soak the foods in a dilute food grade hydrogen peroxide mixture for at least twenty minutes, and then wash it off. This is really important if you are eating produce raw, as in salads. To minimize *"POPs"*, choose organically grown yields, instead. Yes, they are more expensive, but what value are you going to put on your continuing good health? It's priceless, isn't it?

Avoid Genetically Modified Foods

In the USA there are 5 crops that are always Genetically Modified. They are Sugar Beets, Corn, Soya, Cotton (not likely to eat it!) and Rapeseed. In Europe, the story is a little different, but an EU Vote in January 2015 allowed the Member States to decide for themselves. Britain, it seems, is to go ahead and introduce GM corn. Genetically Modified organisms are created by taking genes from entities like bacteria, viruses or animals and insects and then inserting these foreign genes into what is often an unrelated species. Pesticides (POPs) can be implanted into crops themselves, which supposedly makes the plants impervious to parasites. There have been far too many unanswered questions relating to the overall safety of this controversial farming technique. In the USA, the world leader in this technology, it is not required for producers to mark foods as "Genetically Modified". Clearly, this protects brand leaders like Monsanto and DuPont. Soya is the most common GM crop. If you buy any soy-related product that originates in America there is a very good chance it has been modified. This includes isolates and soya protein which are much favored by athletes and bodybuilders the world over. **Unless you can be genuinely sure your soy protein powder has not been genetically altered, don't buy it**.

Xenoestrogens

They come to us via insecticides, fungicides and pesticides which have an estrogen effect. About 2,600 cases of invasive breast cancer will be diagnosed in men in 2016 in the USA. What is shocking is that the incidence of male breast cancer has risen significantly over the last 40 years. Here is the real brain frizzle, 90% of those breast cancers are ER positive. ER stands for "*Estrogen Receptor*". As with female breast cancer, it's often not natural estrogen that is causing the cancer, but *xenoestrogens* which are foreign invaders posing as estrogen. These phony estrogens form because of long-term exposure to toxins that can be found in.....commercial meats and dairy products, vegetables that have been sprayed with insecticides, unfiltered tap water (**NEVER DRINK TAP WATER**), products that contain *paraben* (preservatives found in cosmetics, body care products and pharmaceuticals), *phenoxyethanol* which is glycol ether used as a preservative, plastic packing material treated with *phthalates* (used in plastic products to make them more flexible), using plastic wrap, plastic containers and Styrofoam in the microwave (**THROW AWAY YOUR MICROWAVE**), foods that contain artificial additives and sweeteners as well as canned foods that contain *bisphenol-A* (BPA).

Soya

Soy has been touted as a health product ever since the Second World War. This is more the work of advertising agencies than of pure science. Soya is naturally high in glutamate. You find glutamate in *MSG*. Neurosurgeon Dr. Russel Blaylock urges us to forget about the monosodium, but instead focus on the fact that anything that contains glutamate is an *"excitotoxin"*, which kills brain cells. The problem does not stop with the brain; there are glutamate receptors everywhere in the body; these stimulate the growth of cancer cells. Next time you visit an Asian restaurant be sure to inform the waiter you want no *MSG* in your food. According to Dr. Blaylock cancer cells thrive on two main foods; glutamine and sugar! Of the two he reckons glutamine is worse. That is not the end of the story, however, because Soya contains a load of other toxins, which include aluminum, fluoride and manganese. The wheel rolls full circle when we go back to plant based estrogens. We have talked about the effect of Xenoestrogens on men and how this has caused a rise in the seemingly unlikely problem of breast cancer. Incidentally, male sperm counts have also dropped by over 50% in the last half century. This is a related topic and nobody is talking about it! However, estrogen is a hormone we more commonly relate with women and clever advertising has increased the demand for "soya-based" diet products, particularly amongst women whom it most affects! The result has been that the many females who are already estrogen dominant are ingesting, even more estrogen. This has caused them to have more difficult periods, infertility levels have augmented whilst cases of *PCOS* (polycystic ovarian syndrome) have soared. Post-menopausal women might need a touch more estrogen but everybody else probably doesn't, certainly not men! **CUT BACK ON SOYA, IF NOT EXCLUDE IT!**

Canola Oil

This cooking oil is heavily marketed as a healthy choice. Is it? I think the answer is definitely *"no"*. Canola is made from rapeseed; that yellow crop that spreads all over southern England in the summer! It looks pretty, but cows won't eat it! They know it contains poison. They might not understand the poison is called "ERUCIC ACID" and it contains *"GLUCOSINOLATES*. They give rapeseed an unpleasantly bitter taste. Since 1995 Monsanto has been genetically modifying rapeseed in North America by implanting their weed-killer *"Roundup"* in the plant. The name Canola was registered as a trademark in 1970. The CAN stands for Canada where it originated and OLA is a variant of the word oil. Because of the poisons and the taste, the crop has to be refined before it can be bottled and sold off in grocery stores. The refining process is very different from the cold press method used In Olive Oil; it looks far from natural. **AVOID CANOLA**; use instead cold pressed Olive and Coconut Oils which have not been heated or processed with toxic hexane.

Aspartame

Here's an example of another *"excitotoxin"*. How this

product is allowed to be sold on the open market simply beats me! The chemical was developed by Donald Rumsfeld's, *"G.D. Searle Pharmaceutical Company"*. They first developed the powder as a medicine when they were looking for an inhibitor to the gastrointestinal secretory hormone gastrin, meaning it was invented to serve as an anti-acid. During the process, some of the powder spilled on the researcher's work table and he absent-mindedly tasted it; it was sweet! That's how aspartame, was born. It was first mentioned in *"The Journal of the American Chemical Society"* in 1969; Searle got it on the market as a food and not a pharmaceutical medicine as that was a lot easier. When they first began sales, they described it as being 200 sweeter than sugar and incidentally much cheaper! Later they sold the formula to Monsanto for a huge profit. Today you will find it under the trade names *"Nutra-Sweet"* and *"Equal"*. Aspartame is used in dozens of foods as a sugar substitute, whilst millions of people all over the world use it to sugar-coat their coffee or consume it in *"diet"* related soft drinks like *"Coke Zero"*. Aspartame is a compound containing methanol (wood alcohol). This is used in the production of formaldehyde, an embalming fluid; it is also utilized to dilute petroleum products during the manufacture of gasoline. Aspartame also contains phenylalanine (amino acid) along with aspartic acid (another excitotoxin). All those ingredients make your sugar replacement a carcinogen. Another interesting finding that completely debunks the weight loss claims of Aspartame is it and glutamate burn out leptin receptors. Leptin is the hormone that suppresses appetite. The diet soda that asserts it is there to help you lose weight, is lying to you. Instead, it increases inflammation and encourages weight gain by stimulating your appetite. This is a very dangerous substance. **AVOID ASPARTAME AT ALL COSTS.**

Smoking

Cigarette smoke contains over 4000 chemicals. The mix includes 43 known carcinogens as well as 400 other poisons. The toxic conglomeration includes benzenes, cadmium (a heavy metal), our friend formaldehyde, hydrogen cyanide (they used it to gas inmates at Auschwitz), lead (an all pervasive heavy metal), nickel (some believe this to play a big part in the development of breast and prostate cancer), toluene as well as the powerful addictive agent nicotine. Cigarette smoking hugely increases inflammation. *Why would you want to willingly place any of these toxins into your body?* Smoking as well as inhaling other people's used smoke is an open invitation to free radical damage. If you are a smoker….**STOP RIGHT NOW.** Stopping smoking is the most important health gift you can give to yourself. There is no point in continuing with the remainder of "A Cat Has Nine Lives And So Do You" until you have stopped. Contact us and we'll work with you to help you QUIT.

healthambitconsultancy@protonmail.com

Alcohol

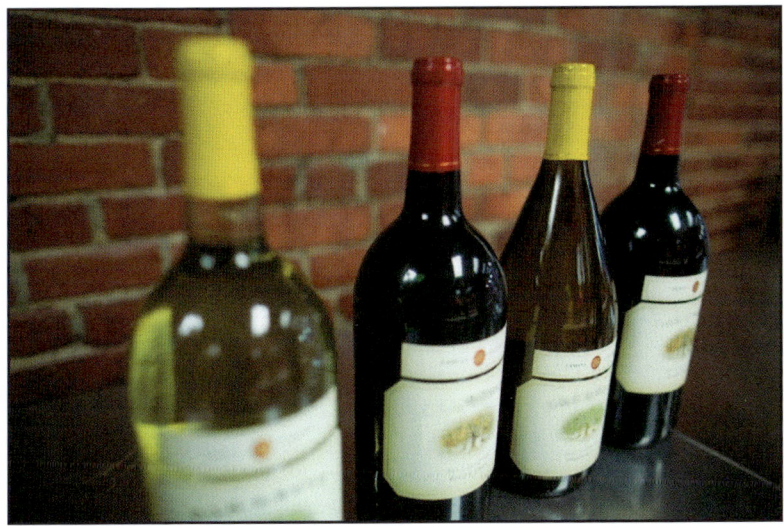

Alcohol weakens the immune system and causes nutritional deficiencies. From an immune standpoint, it decreases the number of white blood cells. When white blood cells die, killer white cells decrease too, meaning macrophages are affected, making it difficult for them to come up with tumor necrosis factor. This is a very negative scenario in the case of cancer. Alcohol is effectively sugar, any word ending in "ol" is a sugar. That means all the cautions applying to sugar also relate to alcohol. Most wines contain sulfates and sulfites. The sulfites come from the soil. They are frequently added as preservatives to the must. They have often been combined again after fermentation to prevent the wines re-fermenting. They are helpful during the wine making process, they offer scant value afterwards, often imparting undesirable taste qualities. Many people have allergic reactions to them as well. No wine is truly sulfite-free, but some come very low in Sulfur. "Chateau Le Puy Cotes de Francs" is a Bordeaux which provides a good example of such a wine. Low Sulfur wines, though, do prove to be a bit on the pricey side. By the way, sulfites are anti-oxidants, so a glass or two of a good red wine helps in your battle against inflammation. Studies show light drinking to be OK, but heavy imbibing is quite another story. How light is daily light? Quite light I am afraid. Beer = half pint, Wine (preferably red) = 1 medium glass, Spirits = 1 measure. 3 or more drinks are likely to make you drunk. **Always drink with caution**.

Weight loss

According to wellness expert Dr. Norman Shealy: *"The instance of overweight and pure and simple obesity has doubled in the last thirty years. People who truly are obese by medical definition are those with a body mass index of 30 or above. That means if you're forty pounds or more above your ideal maximum weight, you're obese, pure fact. And that is equal to the risk of smoking two packs of cigarettes per day, it knocks a hunk off your life."* If your BMI (Body Mass Index) is 25 or above, you are overweight. Of course, if you are a body builder or a super fit athlete carrying a lot of muscle this caveat does not apply. Why? Muscle weighs more than fat. "A Cat Has Nine Lives And So Do You," is designed to assist your weight loss. The 1 Week "Herbal Detox Program" would definitely be the way to go if weight loss is your principal target. Come back to us and we'll schedule a cost free *"weight Loss conversation"* to help you on your way. You can e-mail:

healthamabitconsultancy@protonmail.com

...to set up the call. How do you know you are overweight? A simple way to find out is to calculate your BMI. There is an easy formula. This one is metric. 1) Divide your weight in Kilograms by your height in Meters. 2) Then divide the answer by your height to get the BMI. If you weigh 76 Kgs and your height is 174

Centimeters here's an example of how to do the math. 76 -:- 174 = 0.43678 =:= 174= 25.1. Much easier though to use one of the tables which you can find on the internet.

These on-line calculators work for metric and pounds, so all differences are catered for with the exception of the British Isles who work in stones. One stone=14 lbs. For you, there is a conversion table which works in lbs., kilograms and stones. Ask Mr. Google to help you find this conversion app.

The Benefits of Good Breathing

Breathing detoxifies. The body is designed to release 70% of its toxins through deep breathing. If you are not breathing effectively the other organs are working under increased pressure to make up for the default. If the *"detox"* system is under pressure there is a greater likelihood of *"dis-ease"* occurring. Recent studies have demonstrated that on inhaling most people take in air that has an oxygen content of 20%. The outbreath contains 16% oxygen, meaning that only 4% of the available oxygen has been absorbed. Oxygen is essential for the production of energy. This experiment shows there is a 96% difference between the maximum energetic potential and the actual potential. That is a staggering difference. The lesson is clear. We all need to learn to breathe better. It's essential the inhaled oxygen enters the bloodstream. To achieve this slow, rhythmic and complete breathing is crucial. Blood requires good hemoglobin. That's the protein molecule in red blood cells that carries oxygen from the lungs and returns carbon dioxide from the tissues back to the lungs. Hemoglobin comprises 4 protein molecules connected together in a globulin chain. This chain contains an iron-containing porphyrin called heme. Embedded in the heme is a single atom of iron. This plays a starring role in the transportation of oxygen and carbon dioxide. It is also responsible for giving blood its red color. Quality hemoglobin requires good and healthy nutrition. This fixes the oxygen in place, without it, you have a big problem. You can take iron supplements to fix anemia; except in emergencies, it is never a good idea. Besides for iron to be truly absorbed it must come from an organic source. The same applies to other metals (minerals) too. You can't chew on a lump of iron, it has to come in an assimilatable manner, meaning it needs to be present in our food. Red meat is a good supplier but so are many fruit and vegetables which absorb the iron from the earth. Best then to get iron supplies from natural foods like beetroot, black cherries, green leafy veggies and spirulina. Spirulina, a freshwater alga is easily digested; it contains 28 times more iron than beef liver. Chlorophyll also activates the production of hemoglobin. The reason is the two are remarkably similar. Chlorophyll can be described as the blood of plants. Instead of having an iron atom at its center, it has Magnesium. Vegetables are chock full of chlorophyll, it gives them their green color. However, the very best source is wheatgrass. Wheatgrass juice is deliciously sweet and you don't need a lot. It truly packs the punches. 30ml of wheatgrass juice carries the nutritional equivalent of more than 2 kilos of the best raw organic vegetables according to the renowned Hippocrates Health Institute. A wheatgrass shot on an empty stomach helps cleanse the liver as well as the blood. It packs the body full of healing sunshine. If you've never tried it, do so. Beware, though, you could become addicted!

You Need to Breathe Through Your Nose

In order to oxygenate, always remember the crucial importance of exercise. But there is more and you may not know it! Through breathing, you open up the blood vessels, increase the airways and most importantly switch off the sympathetic mode of the Autonomic Nervous System. This is the stress response, or adrenal dominated" *flight and fight*". When stressed experts urge you to breathe deeply. Many authorities have got it wrong. Dr. Konstantin Buteyko, the originator of the breathing method that bears his name emphasizes we need to breathe through the nose and breathe less. The nose has over 30 functions. It filets and warms the air we breathe but it also releases Nitric Oxide; this sterilizes the air and opens up the airways so more oxygen is transported to the blood. Nitric Oxide helps with heart conditions. Nitroglycerin was often prescribed for those with angina because it increases the level of blood oxygen. Nitroglycerin releases Nitric Oxide! Amongst many other attributes *"NO"* is renowned for reducing inflammation. To achieve this end it is essential we all become *"nose breathers"* and not *"mouth breathers"*. Studies have shown that 50% of children are mouth breathers, and possibly they continue the practice as they grow-up and become adults. Which are you? Clue... if you have ever suffered from asthma, have crooked teeth or snore, chances are you are a mouth breather. Snoring interferes with restful sleep and causes fatigue. Solution: become a *"nose breather"*. Breathe through the nose and breathe less. When you start doing this you will notice your body temperature increases. Your hands and feet become nice and warm, too. This is a sign that you have switched off the sympathetic mode of the autonomic nervous system. When you are stressed, you are in sympathetic dominance which is a left over from the days we used to live in caves and were threatened by dangerous animals like saber tooth tigers. When confronted by a fearsome beast we can *"run away"* or *"fight"* it. The third option is to *"freeze"* and do nothing in the hopes it will pass you by. Not always a good idea! In order to run or fight, adrenaline triggers the body to enter a *"super"* state where you are stronger and quicker. For instance blood shifts from hands and feet into deeper muscle so you can run faster or if the tiger bites you, the bleeding will be less. Cold hands and feet are a sure sign of stress. Now, let's turn the stress switch off through breathing. Place one hand on your chest and the other on your navel. Breathe in through your nose very gently, your chest does not enlarge, it's your stomach that does the work. Notice the colder air coming in and the warmer air leaving. Breathe in gently on the count of 7, hold the breath for the count of 7 and then breathe out on the count of 14. You will see you feel a little breathless. Repeat this exercise nine times. You should feel increased body temperature. That's a sure sign you have exited *"flight and fight"*. It's useful to repeat the exercise before eating, as stress knocks out digestion and before sleeping. Try it and see.

More about Flight and Fight!

It was Professor John Newport Langley who first coined the phrase *"autonomic nervous system"*; this was in 1903. He identified three parts: sympathetic, parasympathetic and enteral (referring to the intestinal system). His discovery revealed the phenomenon of *"Flight and Fight"*. When stressed the system has two related reactions; run away or stay and fight. The response trigger is the overdrive hormone *"adrenaline"*. The purpose is to overcome the perceived threat. Blood pressure increases, blood flow is diverted from surface capillaries to deep muscle, eyesight is improved and systems like digestion and reproduction, all unnecessary and energy consuming functions are switched off for the duration of the emergency. When the danger is passed, top gear becomes unnecessary and a more restful parasympathetic is selected. Now, homeostasis is restored, so you can put your feet up, have dinner and then doze off into a peaceful sleep. Today the chance of bumping into a hungry lion whilst out shopping is extremely slight. But people are more stressed than ever before. What's going on? Sadly biology hasn't kept pace with technology. When the *"Flight and Fight"* response first evolved, man existed in a much slower age. He was a hunter, lived in a cave and came across a life-threatening event on an occasional basis; perhaps once every three weeks. Today there are very few genuine life or death situations. We are all geared up to the horrendous dangers of terrorism, which we are told puts everyone's life at risk, but The March, 2011, *Harper's* Index noted:

*The Number of American civilians who died worldwide in terrorist attacks last year: 8 — Minimum number who died after being struck by lightning: 29.*It seems there are overall far fewer threats to life today than there were in the past. We are responding to non-life threatening situations as if they were death provoking. These situations come fast and furious. Several inappropriate reactions can and often do take place during the course of an average day. There is no time for the body to recover. The adrenals get tired, the digestive system closes down, and so does reproduction. This leaves the liver overwhelmed as it mops up all the chemicals that have been released by a sympathetic perceived response to non-life threatening events. Threats include a row with the wife, an encounter with the boss at work, or some driver cutting you up on the street. Yes, road rage is a flight or fight reaction! What's the solution? You've got it, nose breathing using the simple exercise above. It can't get any better than that, can it?

The Crucial Importance of Sleep

Every one of us requires between 7 and 8 hours of restful sleep every night. There are few exceptions to the rule. Margaret Thatcher boasted she could make do with only 4. But was she human? Dr. Norm Shealy has this to say: *"Dying is not a big deal, but dwindling for 20-30 years with multiple diseases is to me torture!"* Insomnia is a very common health problem. It weakens the immune system, contributes to obesity, diabetes and heart disease and causes a tremendous heap of human suffering that can lead to old-age hell. If sleep is a problem for you, now is the time to address the issue. Supplementing with the mineral Magnesium has proved to be an outstanding solution. Magnesium is *"Nature's de-stressor"*. This alkaline substance soothes the body, calms the nerves as well as promoting sound sleep. Spinach, black beans, halibut and pumpkin seeds all provide good sources. However, when it comes to sleeplessness, taking a supplement is the preferred option. Take 1000mg daily, preferably in two 500mg doses, one in the morning and the second just before bed. The most bioavailable form is Magnesium Chloride; it's super soluble in water. Acid complexes and their sub-sets involving amino acid chelation are also well absorbed. This type of Magnesium relies for its efficiency not on solubility but on protein pathways. Magnesium amino acid chelates include Magnesium Glycinate (possibly the best), Magnesium Lysinate, Magnesium Orotate and Magnesium Taurate. Because of the complex chemical processes involved in their production; they tend to be the most expensive. Melatonin is another natural sleep enhancer (a hormone made by the pineal gland) It helps control the sleep and wake cycle. During daytime the pineal is inactive, but it livens up after sunset. Then it starts releasing Melatonin into the bloodstream. Levels rise sharply after 9 pm, you feel less alert as you prepare for sleep. Melatonin supplements enhance this natural sleep affect. Pill strengths vary between 2 and 20mg. In my experience, 3mg nods you off for something like 3 hours. Higher doses may leave you feeling groggy on awakening. It's a brilliant sleep inducer on long distance flights too and helps hugely with jet lag. Sadly Melatonin is not available in EU countries. Another aid is homeopathic Coffea Cruda. Just as coffee revs you up, the homeopathic variant produces the reverse effect, easing many stress-related symptoms, including insomnia due to an overactive mind. I suggest taking a 30C dose on retiring and a further 30c if you should wake up during the night, a first-rate supplier of homeopathic remedies is Ainsworth's Homeopathic Pharmacy, situated at, 36 New Cavendish St, London W1G 8UF. Their phone number is +44 (0) 207 935 5330 or see the website

www.ainsworths.com

The Body's Many Cries for Water

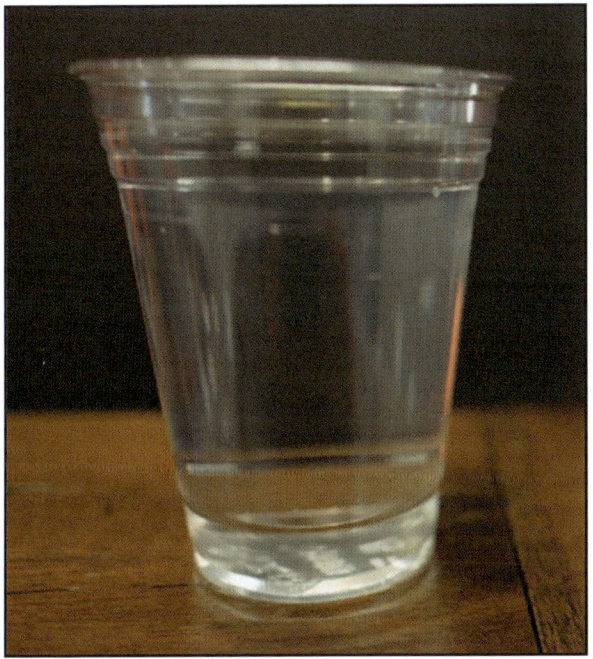

Figure 5

Most people are dehydrated because they don't drink enough water. A myth suggests we should all drink 8 glasses per day. Nobody knows where this came from, so let's ignore it. There is, however, a simple formula. You drink 35ml of water per kilo of body weight. If you weigh 65 kilos you need to drink 2 and a quarter liters of water daily. This is water, other drinks like coffee, tea and juices are over and above that amount. Dr. Fereydoon Batmanghelidj, a British-trained physician, served as the Shah of Iran's personal Doctor. After the Revolution, he was imprisoned in the notorious Evin Prison, under sentence of death. He remained a prisoner for 3 years, during which time he continued his work as a health care practitioner. The authorities refused to give him any medicines, so he used the single resource available to him, water. He is the author of *"Your Body's Many Cries for Water'*. In the book, he writes about his findings. Apparently, thirst is only one way of expressing dehydration. He feels a dry mouth is an advanced stage of lack. His clinical experience in prison gave him the skill to assign several different illnesses which he saw as symptoms of dehydration. This broad list of maladies includes asthma, angina, indigestion and obesity. In Chapter 5 of his book he makes this amazing statement: *"Pathology that is seen to be associated with "social stresses" – fear, anxiety, insecurity, persistent emotional and marital problems and the creation of depression- are the results of water deficiency to the point the water requirements of the brain tissue are affected."* Water in preference medication, that's a thought! Don't, however, drink tap water, it's full of impurities, and plastic bottles pose many problem, too. For starters they take up to 400 years to decompose; we have an ecological disaster in the making. The plastic contains phthalates, these are xenoestrogens and we've discussed them already. Another worrying factor is the acidification of water. It is supposed to be a neutral point between acids and alkalines with a pH of 7. Over acidity is a key to disease. When blood and other fluids lean towards a more alkaline level, illness is inhibited. Besides blood pH has a very narrow window of opportunity; it lies between 7.36 and 7.45 with an average of 7.41 When pH drops to the lower end of the scale, acidosis occurs whilst we have alkalosis at the higher end. If the blood becomes too acid it is a life threatening event. The system tries to correct the crisis by drawing alkalizing calcium from bones, as this happens the bones are weakened. That is one of the principal causes of osteoporosis. Drink water, then, that is alkaline. Certain brands of bottled water have acceptably high levels. Evian water comes out at a reasonable 7.2 whilst Fiji water racks up an amazing score of 7.7. You can help the process yourself by adding a slice of lime or lemon. These fruits have an acid pH outside the body, but inside they become highly alkaline. Usually with a pH in the region of 8. This is a cheaper option than buying expensive waters imported from half-way across the globe. Better still purchase a high-quality water filter; then your plastic bottle problem is also solved. Many people used to advise avoiding drinking water during meals. New evidence shows that mealtime dehydration stresses the liver particularly if the food is salty and the digestive system lacks bicarbonate. By all means, drink room temperature water during eating, but avoid ice water as Chinese Medicine warns us, it puts out the digestive fire. If your goal is weight loss, drink a large glass half an hour before eating as it will curb your appetite.

Are Nutritional Supplements Worthwhile?

There is a lot of controversy surrounding nutritional supplements. Many Doctors claim they are totally unnecessary because you can get all the vitamins and minerals required from food. Anyone who makes this claim is utterly detached from reality. Intensive farming methods and artificial fertilizers like NPK have leached the goodness from the soil. We have touched on this already. Farming is now an industry and the farmers want the earth to produce higher yields to increase their profits. Traditionally fields were allowed to lie fallow in order for the soil to rest and replete itself, but not anymore. This has diminished the vitamin and mineral quality of the earth itself, and this lack has reflected itself by way of a depletion of vital nutrients in the human diet. What's the answer? As we have already stressed, wherever possible buy organic products. Yes, above and beyond that, you do need to take first-rate supplements, not the cheaper varieties that appear on supermarket shelves. It is always worth remembering that you get what you pay for. Quality comes with a price tag! I regard supplements as medicines and they really need to come from a natural source to yield the best results. Basically, everybody needs to take a quality multi-vitamin and mineral pill daily, plus a reliable source of anti-oxidants to fight inflammation. Ascorbic

Acid masquerades as Vitamin C. It is made cheaply in a laboratory, true Vitamin C derives from a natural, plant based source like rose hips or acerola. Both varieties will sacrifice electrons to arrest the mad rampage of electrons that have somehow become de-partnered. Both types yield results but for the best results, I recommend you buy a product containing synergistic bio-flavonoids. If you are unsure on what brand to purchase, enlist the help of a knowledgeable assistant in your local health food store.

The Vital Importance of Vitamin D

Vitamin D is a fat-soluble vitamin that mimics a hormone in some ways. It's important because it plays a starring role in how the body manages calcium. It does this by keeping it in its proper place and moving it on so it does not stick to the side of arteries as plaque. "D" strengthens teeth and bones; essential in childhood. This amazing vitamin protects against muscle weakness as well as giving protection against the hormone-related cancers like breast and prostate. Vitamin D enhances thyroid function, boosts the immune response, helps soothe arthritis and aids the blood in clotting efficiently. D-25-hydroxyvitamin D-3 is usually used as the marker. D-2 (ergocalciferol), originates from a food source, D-3 (cholecalciferol) comes from sunlight; there is a synthetic variety identified as D-5. Of these variants, experts consider D-3 the best choice. Ultra-Violet B rays from the sun stimulate the body to make vitamin D-3 in the skin because of a reaction with cholesterol. Commercial sunscreens filter out the UV-B light because it causes sunburn in excess. Sadly this also prevents the synthesis of life-enhancing Vitamin D. Don't slap on the sunscreen, instead expose yourself to between 15 and 20 minutes of strong sunlight at least three times per week. After that go ahead and apply a protective agent. This pre-supposes you live somewhere the sun actually shines! People living north of 30* latitude or south of the same are likely to be sun-deprived, especially during the winter months; meaning they will be unable to make enough Vitamin D to ensure good health. You have a choice, either move to a sunnier clime or start supplementing. Buy your Vitamin D-3 in a minimum pill strength of 1000 IU. You will need to take a minimum of 1500 IU daily; this is the very basic requirement. Sometimes the dose will have to be a lot higher than that. The current RDA of 400 IU is useless! A study published in *"The New England Journal of Medicine"* demonstrated that a deficiency amongst older adults was widespread. 57% of older people showed up with dangerously low levels of Vitamin D. The investigating team felt this was a major reason why osteoporosis is such a threat to this age group. Apart from the healing of the sun's rays, Vitamin D is found in cod liver oil, mackerel, dairy products along with eggs, butter, shitake mushrooms, salmon, sardines and sweet potatoes. Liver and Gallbladder disorders interfere with Vitamin D absorption. Anybody in that category needs to be very careful.

Oil Pulling

Also known as *"Kavala"*, where the oil is swished around the mouth or *"gundusha"* where it's simply held there. This is an ancient Ayurvedic health technique. You take a couple of teaspoons of extra-virgin Coconut Oil into your mouth and then *"swish"* it around for between ten and twenty minutes. The practice is best performed first thing in the morning before eating anything. This *"swishing"* or *"oil pulling"* has multiple benefits; it eliminates toxins and bacteria, which are taken up by the oil. After twenty minutes you spit it out which over the time has taken on the consistency of water. Don't swallow this, spit it out and then rinse out your mouth with water, which you expel, too. Timing is important as twenty minutes allows the oil to break-up plaque and bacteria but not long enough for the body to start reabsorbing the toxins. Coconut Oil is a natural *"bacteriostatic agent"*, it has a pleasant taste and it kills streptococcus mutans, the bacteria known to create dental caries according to the British Dental Journal. The process assists in whitening teeth, whilst *de-toxing* the system. *The de-tox* effect can cause mild congestion along with slight headaches as the mucous drains from the sinus cavities. Fear not, it will quickly pass. My personal experience has been extremely positive as oil pulling has eliminated gingivitis and bleeding gums. It still brings up mucous, but isn't this one of the remarkable methods of expelling toxins? However, you need to be patient, results may not be immediate but they will come. Coconut Oil is an effective breath freshener and much preferable to a chemical mouth-wash. The stuff becomes solid at temperatures lower than 23C. Don't be put off when confronted with a *"lump"*; it quickly melts in the mouth. If that's unpleasant, warm it, which liquefies it. Dr. Bruce Fife is arguably the foremost expert on Coconut Oil, In his book, *"Oil Pulling Therapy"*, he says *"Some people think I'm crazy when I tell them that oil pulling can help with asthma, allergies, chronic fatigue, diabetes, migraine headaches, PMS as well as chronic skin problems. Oil pulling works by detoxifying or cleansing the body. In this way disease promoting toxins are removed, thus allowing the body to heal itself. As a consequence health problems of all types improve."* Try it and see for yourself!

The Magic of Dark Chocolate

Now for a treat: *"Chocolate the food of the Gods"*, that's how the Aztecs described it! Chocolate has some astonishing health benefits; I am not talking about sugar-laden milk chocolate. Raw cacao is not sweet, it's bitter, that's because of all the polyphenols it contains. "Polyphenols" is a generic term for several thousand plant based molecules which are chock full of inflammation-fighting anti-oxidants. I think by now you are starting to get the picture which is the more anti-oxidants the better. Cacao is the main ingredient in chocolate making. It's not the pods but the dried seeds, also known as nibs that make-up the raw material. If you are a purist in search of maximum health benefits, then it's nibs that you are looking for. Their bitter taste puts some people off, but they can be ground up and included in smoothies which make them more pleasant. If this is too much for you; choose chocolate itself. *"Good chocolate"* is high in cacao and low in sugar. Select a product with a cacao content in excess of 70%, but 85% would be much better. You can find chocolate as high as 99% cacao, but a little of that goes a long way. Why is cacao so good? Its benefits relate to several naturally occurring compounds. These include *epicatechin* (a flavonoid which acts as a formidable anti-oxidant).This is a phytonutrient that is widely used in Chinese and Ayurvedic medicine affording skin protection, brain enhancement and blood pressure regulation. Much nicer to eat chocolate than take a beta-blocker! Another compound is *Resveratrol*. Another potent anti-oxidant that is powerful enough to cross the blood-brain barrier and subsequently dispels inflammation in the Central Nervous System. In 2012, a study showed that eating dark chocolate could slash the risk of cardiovascular disease by 37% and reduce stroke risk by 29%. Another meta-analysis in the same year showed chocolate lowered insulin resistance, reduced blood pressure, whilst increasing the elasticity of blood vessels as well as slightly reducing LDL cholesterol levels. An article in *"The Journal of Oxidative Medicine and Cellular Longevity"* said: *"Cocoa contains about 380 known chemicals which are psychoactive compounds. …..It has more phenolics and higher anti-oxidant capacity than green tea, black tea or red wine. The phenolics from cocoa may protect against diseases in which oxidative stress is implicated as a causal or contributing factor such as cancer."* Here's a treat, eat dark chocolate with a cacao content of 85% or more. You can't eat too much as the flavor is too rich. Besides, it provides an excellent source of Magnesium.

Apples

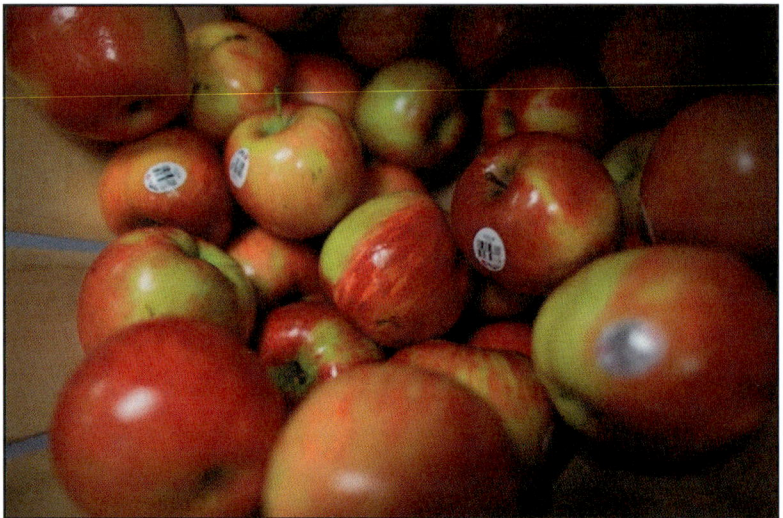

Figure 6

Apples synergize the beneficial effects of dark chocolate. It's simply delicious to eat them together.

The Benefits of Sea Salt

Current research refutes earlier studies extolling the virtues of how low salt diets reduce high blood pressure. Dr. Axe claims it's not salt but the type of salt that causes the problem. The devil is in the detail; it looks as if the devil comes in the form of commercially produced *"table salt"*. The manufacturing process strips the product of all its naturally occurring minerals. They take sea salt, heat it to 650*C which equates to 1200*F. The residue that materializes from such aggressive heat exposure is 97.5% Sodium Chloride and a 2.5% miscellany of other ingredients, which include anti-caking agents, Iodine to prevent goiters, MSG (an excitotoxin) to help stabilize the Iodine and aluminum derivatives like solo-co-aluminate. Conversely sea salt contains more than 60 trace minerals, they assist hydration and provide sufficient Sodium to create a balance with Potassium. The minerals contain powerful electrolytes like Magnesium and produce trace elements to insure correct adrenal, immune and thyroid function as well as producing some digestive enzymes. Doesn't that sound like a better mix? Moreover, sea salt is an alkalyser, a blood sugar balancer, an eliminator of mucous, an immune system assistant, an electrolyte stabilizer, a sleep aid, whilst it prevents muscle cramps, it acts as a heart rate and blood pressure regulator and what's more it makes food taste better! Isn't that a perfect mix? Sea salt is preferable to Himalayan Rock salt which contains iron, giving it its pinkish color. Excessive iron creates problems, like exacerbating prostate difficulties, and a reaction with Vitamin C that is a cause for heart conditions. Dr. Hal Huggins points out all inorganic minerals produce a residue that when combined with excessive blood lipids manufacture arterial plaque. It's always a good idea to go easy on the salt, even sea salt.

Smoothies an Ideal Way to Eat the Rainbow

Smoothies make a delicious breakfast. You can put lots of healthy fruit and vegetables into the blender and easily achieve the daily target of seven or more servings. Here are some tips: 1) Have a juice base. I use apple or coconut. 2) Now add a handful of berries 3) 1 banana 4) 1 small cucumber 5) a handful of parsley 6) a clove of garlic 7) a teaspoon of turmeric 8) a teaspoon of Coconut Oil 9) A tablespoon of live yogurt 10) 1 raw egg 11) a generous pinch of black pepper 12) an apple 13) a small teaspoon of ascorbic acid and anything else that catches your fancy. That will provide a very generous smoothie, probably sufficient for two people. That version has five fruit and veg servings which go a long way towards your 7 or more portions. It's just a suggestion. Now go ahead and create your own. Tony Robbins used to say: *"sell your car and buy a juicer"*.

Juicers are for juices and blenders are for smoothies. And cars….that's another story!

Yes, buy fresh wheat grass or grow your own and juice a good daily measure. A shot of wheatgrass contains the goodness of 2 kilos of fresh vegetables, so it must count as a serving on its own. The question people frequently ask is what is a serving? 1 apple = 1 serving, 1 orange = 1 serving, 7-8 strawberries = 1 serving, a small bowl of spinach = 1 serving, 1 large banana = 1 serving, 150 ml of fresh vegetable juice = 1 serving.

There are many kinds of juicers on the market. The best juicer is one you will use! Some are complex and difficult to clean. You might not use one of those for very long. Cheap juicers are centrifugal. They have a fast rotating blade that breaks down the fruit or vegetable. They encourage juice flow, but the heat they create damages the enzymes. That means you have to drink the juice soon after it is made. It will not store because of the enzyme kill off. More expensive slow juicers don't cause a heat problem. That allows you to store the juice in the fridge. The problem with juice is it contains very little fiber. We all need to intake between 30-50 mg of fiber every day. Smoothies contain fiber which makes them a better option.

Green Tea versus Coffee

A cup of good quality, non-instant coffee without sugar and milk is an excellent health drink. It assists with bathrooms visits and it does contain anti-oxidants, but it also contains large quantities of caffeine. A little is good but a lot is not! Tea is considered to be the most consumed beverage in the world after water, but most of it is black tea. Green tea is produced from the un-oxidized leaves of the *Camellia sinensis* bush. It is less processed than the black variety so it is able to keep most of the anti-oxidants and beneficial polyphenols found in the raw product. Traditional Chinese and Ayurvedic medicine use green tea to control bleeding and aid in wound healing. However, it's also useful in aiding digestion, improving heart conditions, recovering mental health as well as regulating body temperature. A cup of green tea provides an excellent after dinner digestive aid, much better than coffee. According to the National Cancer Institute, the polyphenols in green tea have shown to decrease tumor growth in animal lab tests. Countries where green tea consumption is high, have lower cancer rates. One large clinical study compared green tea drinkers with non-drinkers and discovered that those who drank the most tea were less likely to develop pancreatic cancer; in women, this rate was as high as 50%. A 2006 study published in *JAMA* (Journal of the American Medical Association) concluded that green tea consumption *"is associated with reduced mortality due to all causes, including cardiovascular disease......participants who drank at least 5 cups of green tea per day had a significantly lower risk of dying (especially from cardiovascular disease) than those who drank less than one cup of tea a day."* Conclusion swap your coffee for green tea if you would like to enjoy these health benefits.

The Dangers of Sodium Fluoride

Neurosurgeon, Dr. Russel Blaylock in his report *"Why Fluoride is Toxic"*, claims the Authorities are deliberately lying when they declare fluoride to be safe because they carefully ignore the copious scientific evidence to the contrary. One area of research illustrates its apparent part in triggering early onset brain diseases like Alzheimer's. It does this by combining with metals such as aluminum. One specific study confirmed that adding fluoride to water in the presence of small amounts of aluminum resulted in the destruction of cells in the part of the brain controlling learning and memory. It seems fluoride dumbs us down, which is in keeping with anecdotal evidence claiming it was initially used by the Nazis to subdue the prison population in camps like Auschwitz and Bergen-Belsen. The more recent evidence comes from a 1988 study published in the peer-reviewed Journal *"Brain Research"*. But we have been taught that fluoride is essential for preserving dental health. Again current practice flies in the face of facts. There have been numerous studies that conclusively prove fluoride does not reduce dental cavities. So why are the relevant Authorities so concerned with giving us a different story? A 2014 article in *"The Lancet"* accused it of being a neurotoxin in the same category as Mercury, Lead and Arsenic. Although the FDA has banned fluorine-based chemicals in food packaging on grounds of toxicity, it continues to support the Municipal fluoridation of water. Frankly, none of this makes any sense. The message is clear: STOP USING FLUORIDE....That means stop using fluoride-containing toothpaste. There are fluoride-free brands on the market, also refuse to purchase bottled water containing fluoride. Many reputable brands are fluoride- free, notably Evian, Vittel and Volvic or do your own research. Most commercially produced water filters do not remove fluoride. Why? Because it is negatively charged. Minerals like Calcium, Potassium and Magnesium are positively charged; which means negatively- charged fluoride acts like a magnet and extracts these health producing minerals from the system. Do you see now, why avoiding fluoride is so important? Best check to tell if the tap water in your area is fluoridated, but then you don't drink tap water do you? We've mentioned this before. Besides everything else, tap water, by law, must contain a disinfectant and this is usually a variant of chlorine. This kills gut flora stone dead. For a healthy digestive system, you need to generate good healthy gut bacteria. If you want to go into the tap water issue a little further, you need to know it contains a posse of heavy metals along with other contaminants. London tap water, for example, is recycled sewerage. Yes, it has been cleaned and filtered so as the water company claims it to be 100% pure. But is it? Think what people throw down the *"loo"* aside from pee and poo, antibiotics, birth control pills, anti-depressants, Statin Drugs, NSAIDs, the list is practically endless. If you know anything about homeopathy you know that trace amounts are going to slip through the cleansing process, and trace amounts have a medicinal effect. Do you really want to take the risk?

Epsom Salts, No Home Should be Without Them!

Epsom Salts have amazing health benefits, proving a brilliant way of destressing and detoxifying. Unlike other neutrally occurring salts, Epsom, come from a pure mineral compound containing both Magnesium and Sulphate ($MgSO4$). Whilst the body requires Magnesium Sulphate, it's the skin we need to focus upon. It's the second largest organ of detoxification. It gets rid of toxins, but it can also absorb "good stuff." meaning $MgSO4$ can be absorbed by taking an Epsom Salts bath. Incidentally, the salts are named after the bitter salt springs in Epsom, Surrey, a town better known perhaps for its race course, but this is where the porous chalk of the North Downs meets the non-porous London clay. In excess of 325 bodily enzymes require Magnesium in order to function smoothly. It stimulates nerve and muscle function, limits inflammation, improves blood oxygenation as well as flow. It's a fabulous anti-inflammatory agent that provides pain relief by extracting harmful toxins and balancing levels of Magnesium and Sulfur. Don't take Epsom salts. It's a very harsh laxative, but regular Epsom Salts baths are a wonderful experience. Avoid them, however, if you are pregnant, have a heart condition or have cuts or sunburn. Forty minutes given over to this treat weekly is a detoxing delight that will help you onto the path of wellness quite quickly. Use about 4 tablespoons of the salts for every 25 kilos of body weight. Plan on spending forty minutes in the tub. During the initial 20 minutes toxins will be extracted, you should notice the water changing color. During the second 20 minute time-frame you will start to absorb the Magnesium and Sulphur. Light some candles, play some relaxing music and enjoy this amazingly de-stressing experience. Try and repeat it weekly.

To Fast or not to Fast

Eating less is the key to staying young, claims Russian Doctor.

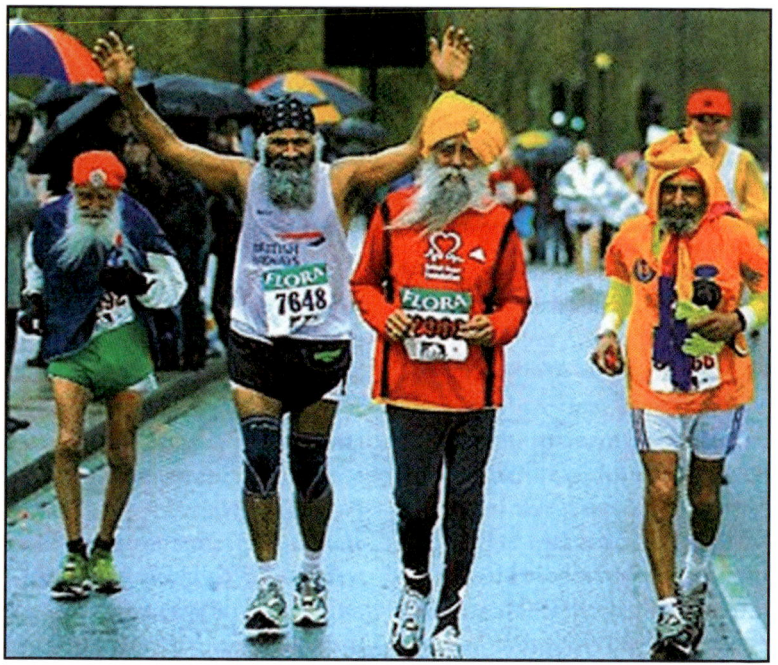

Figure 7

Fauja Singh completed the 2012 London Marathon in seven hours and forty-nine minutes. By no means, a winning time, yet Fauja Singh, affectionately dubbed the *"turbaned tornado"* is 101 years old. He took up long distance running after moving to the UK from his native India; post his wife's death in 1992.

He attributes his long and vigorous life to healthy eating habits. Like most Punjabis he is a strict vegetarian, existing on a diet of lentils, vegetables flavored with ginger, brown bread, fruit and natural yogurt. It's not so much what he eats, but how much! He restricts himself to small, child-sized portions which are reflected in his weight. He is 173 centimeters tall and yet weighs only 53 kilos.

According to Russian-born Dr. Arcady Economo, there is nothing new here. Scientists have known for 80 years that calorie restricted food intake can prolong life. Dr. Clive McCay claimed during the 1930s that such diets could extend life expectancy by up to 50%. Fauja Singh's success in covering the 42 kilometer London Marathon course attests to these claims.

Koh Samui is home to approximately 20 so called "*detox resorts*". They range from the good to the bad and indifferent. They all promote fasting and inner cleansing. People flock from across the globe to these establishments. Some come to embrace better health practices, but most come to lose weight. Dr. Economo runs a group of similar facilities in Hungary and Croatia; his emphasis is on the fasting component of the program. In Budapest and elsewhere his nutritional experts design specific diets for his clients. They are expected to follow these eating programs when they return home after completing their one or two- week detox plan. The most popular of these divides the year into four, thirteen-week blocks. Each chunk comprises one fasting week, with a near zero calorific intake, one recovery week when food is gradually introduced where consumption is limited to 5,200-kilo calories and eleven ordinary weeks. The normal weeks comprise six feeding days calculated at 2,000 calories per day. The seventh day is a fasting day with 0 calories permitted. This formula yields 72 fasting days in the year; it averages out at a usual food input of 1,500 daily calories. It appears Fauja Singh is obtaining the same result simply by eating less on an ongoing basis.

Professor Valter Longo of the University of Southern California's Longevity Institute explains the connection between fasting and increased life span is the hormone "*Insulin Growth Factor-1*". This hormone causes children to develop, but when they reach adulthood it begins to stress the body and appears to cause aging. His evidence is the genetically engineered Laron mouse, which does not produce *IGF-1*. These creatures can live up to five years, much longer than the 2-year life expectancy of a normal mouse. They seem to be immune to cancer and heart disease, and when they die it's because the heart just stops.

Longo goes on to explain that fasting lowers *IGF-1* levels, and when we stop eating the body switches from growth to repair mode when several DNA healing genes switch-on. Dr. Economo feels that eating cessation also reduces damaging free radical levels. The result is a reduction in blood pressure, a decrease in high blood sugar levels, which are in themselves a prelude to diabetes and metabolic levels decrease as the body slows down to conserve its energy resources.

Fasting, especially for the first timer can be difficult. Toxins which are a natural by-product of today's lifestyle release and these can cause headaches, dizziness and a general feeling of unwellness, but if you persevere you're likely to experience extraordinary results! Both Professor Longo and Dr. Economo suggest a prolonged fast is best accomplished under supervision. That comes in the next section of *"A Cat Has Nine Lives And So Do You"*. Stick by and enjoy this guide to longevity, health and wellness.

The A-Z of Longevity, Health and Fitness:

A is for reduced alcohol consumption
B is for breathing through the nose
C is for dark chocolate with 85 % cacao
D is for Don't Smoke
E is for exercise. At least 35 mins daily
F is for free radicals, the cause of inflammation
G is for healthful green tea
H is for health the purpose of all of this!
I is for Instant Coffee- avoid it
J is for juice and juicers
K is for Vitamin K found in green leafy vegetables
L is for laughter. Do it more often
M is magnificent Magnesium, nature's relaxant
N is for Nitric Oxide. It aids the heart; get it through nose breathing

O is for Oxygen so necessary for life
P is for pH. Eat and Drink to be more alkaline
Q is for quiet, we all need quiet time
R is for the rainbow. Be sure to eat it
S is for sugar. Stop it!
T is for Trans Fats. Don't eat them
U is for UVB. The sunshine that makes Vitamin D
V is for Vitamins. We all need them
W is for Water. Drink more of it
X is for Xtra Care. Be sure to take more
Y is for You. You are responsible for your own health
Z is for zzz zzz. Get 8 hours sleep nightly.

Life 1 – The Kidney Cleanse

Let's Begin

Two ever-popular green herbs, rich in vitamins and minerals serve as powerful "kidney cleansers". These are Parsley and Coriander (Cilantro). Both are super effective at removing heavy metals. If you recall from *"the Basics"*, heavy metals play a big part in the creation of inflammation forming free-radicals. We already know Inflammation is the first step on a road that can lead to cancer, heart, kidney and lung disease as well as degenerative bone problems such as osteoporosis.

Studies have shown how Coriander leaves bind to the heavy metals because they contain biochemical magnets that include citric acid, phytic acid and certain electrolytes. The result is an effective free-radical scavenger. It is so powerful that simply placing a bunch of Coriander leaves in a bowl of suspect water can purify it.

Let's not omit Parsley, because it, too, is a potent chelating agent. Like Coriander this herb is full of vitamins and minerals, but it also plays host to "mega" free-radical killer, *"glutathione"*. That's not all; it's an important blood sugar balancer because it protects against insulin resistance. Another important function enjoyed by Parsley is the job it does to remove excess bodily fluids without disturbing potassium levels. As a *"kidney cleanser,"* it eliminates salts along with other mineral solids that have accumulated there. That means it, like Coriander, chelates heavy metals like mercury, cadmium and lead. It's always a sound idea to add this *"dynamic duo"* to salads, foods and morning smoothies. Wait a minute, though. There is more.

How to Make Kidney Cleanse Juice:

Take a large bunch of Coriander or Parsley, or better still combine the two. Place your herbs in a big non-aluminum saucepan. Add a liter of "spring water" (Evian, Volvic or Vittel are fine). Bring the mixture to the boil and then simmer for a further 10 minutes. Turn off the heat and allow to cool. When cool, strain off the leaves and pour the liquid into a glass bottle. Store in the fridge. If the liquid starts to ferment (gets fizzy because it's producing CO_2), that's fine too, because then it becomes a probiotic.

Drink a 50ml shot of the juice, first thing every morning. Be sure it's on an empty stomach! A good idea is to do this before the regular morning oil pulling. For maximum efficiency, I suggest you keep up this practice for 30 days. Afterwards, repeat every 4 months to insure the kidneys are functioning at peak efficiency. Never forget the cleansing power of both Coriander and Parsley, so whether on the cleanse or not be sure to include them regularly in your diet.

Whilst performing the "Kidney Cleanse". It's also highly recommended you supplement with Chlorella. This blue-green alga is high in protein. Studies have shown it to be another strong heavy metal fighter. Combine Chlorella with the *"Kidney Cleanse Juice"* to make an even more effective First Step.

Life 2 – The Mother of All Organs

It's Time to Detox the Gut

Welcome to the world of colonics, enemas and the "Herbal Detox Program." The inventor of *"Cornflakes"* (yes, they were initially marketed as a health food), John Harvey Kellogg said: ***"90% of the diseases of civilization are due to the improper functioning of the bowel."***

When they say *"death begins in the colon"*, *"they"* might be right! Because as Dr. Kellogg suggested, a toxic bowel can contribute to a spate of health complaints. Step 2 of *"A Cat Has Nine Lives And So Do You."* is all about clearing up that mess and asking why was it so toxic in the first place? This article which appeared in "The Guardian" on 9th March 2002 brought me to Koh Samui. It took me a further 4 years, but I got here.

The Enema Within

Ian Belcher took some persuading to go on a colonic irrigation holiday, even at a Thai beach resort. It is, he discovered, quite astonishing what gets flushed out in the course of a week's treatment. But did he feel the better for it?

Ian Belcher
Saturday 9 March 2002

"When photographer Anthony Cullen heard the clank of glass on porcelain, he didn't need to examine the contents of the toilet bowl between his legs. He instinctively knew he had just passed the marble he had swallowed as a five-year-old; the small colored sphere - "I think it was a bluey" - had lodged in his colon for 22 years. His nonchalance was understandable. Having flushed 400 pints of coffee and vinegar solution around his large intestine through 10 enemas, and taken 100 herbal laxatives, he had become hardened to extraordinary sights. He had already excreted yards of long stringy mucus "with a strange yellow glaze", several hard black pellets and numerous pieces of undigested rump steak. Like an iceberg breaking away from a glacier, the marble was simply the latest object to drop off the furred up wall of his colon.

Within 30 minutes it had become a burning topic of conversation among guests at The Spa resort on the Thai island of Koh Samui. Most listened, nodded earnestly and smiled, a flicker of mutual support, before describing their own bowel movements in unnervingly graphic detail. It was just another day at the tropical health farm where conversations that would be deemed unpleasant, if not obscene, in any place outside a gastro-intestinal ward, are mere idle chit-chat among the sun-soaked clientele.

They may have travelled across the world to The Spa's thatched beach huts, encircling its renowned restaurant whose Pod Ka Pow Nam Many Hoy - prawns and chilli, stir-fried in oyster sauce - is a house speciality, but not a morsel of food, nor a single calorie, will pass their lips. Instead they order around 70-odd gallons of coffee and vinegar, lemon or garlic solution - lightly warmed, please waiter - to be squirted up their anus. You are unlikely to find this particular dish on MasterChef.

The roots of their truly alternative activity holiday lie in our modern lifestyle. Some doctors, such as Richard Anderson, inventor of the Clean-Me-Out Programme, claim our high stress existences and over-processed diets - chips, pizzas, burgers - have left us with clogged-up digestive systems. And that, according to advocates of intestinal cleansing, makes us disease time bombs, at increased risk from cancer, heart trouble, infertility, diabetes, premature ageing and, pass the smelling salts this instant, wrinkles.

Their solution is to fast: to put nothing in one end, while simultaneously purifying yourself by propelling significant amounts of liquid up the other. "It's like changing the oil in your car," says Guy Hopkins, the 60-year-old owner of The Spa, whose eyes glint with evangelical zeal when he talks about colonic irrigation. "If you don't do it every so often [your body] isn't going to run that well. We constantly put the wrong fuel in our bodies and, sure, they keep on going, but cleanse yourself and you'll be amazed how much better you'll feel."

A tempting sales pitch, yet when my editor suggested a first-person report, I had grave reservations. As someone whose only concessions to healthy eating had involved switching from butter to olive oil and occasionally cutting the fat off my steak, the fast sounded frankly insane. Then I began hearing about the "lifestyle benefits" of the cleanse, of the 90-degree heat and tropical beaches. Words such as "de-stressing" and "life-changing" were tossed around.

I weakened, dithered and finally relented. The photographer, Anthony, it was agreed, must also fast.

Our preparation began well before we spotted our first palm tree. The Spa recommended we prepared with a fortnight of abstinence from meat, processed foods (adios my daily staples, pasta and bread), milk, cheese, booze, coffee or soft drinks. Instead, our gastric juices were stimulated by salads, fruit, slightly cooked vegetables, herb teas and water.

It wasn't easy. Both Anthony and myself are what might charitably be termed "stocky", enjoying cooking and, more importantly, eating. Within days, food, or lack of it, had become an obsession. We had long phone discussions about interesting ways to grill aubergine; Anthony bragged about his spicy ratatouille. Life was changing.

As the first toxins were expelled and severe caffeine withdrawal set in, I experienced headaches, aching muscles, a lack of energy, and an increasingly short temper. I also faced a new menace: the liver flush drink. Designed to sluice out your system, it's a vile mix of olive oil, raw garlic, and cayenne pepper blended with orange juice. I've no idea if it worked, but my urine turned clear and I always got standing space on the tube.

We stuck rigidly to the diet until disaster struck: an upgrade on the flight to Bangkok. Our willpower collapsed and over the next "lost" 12 hours we demolished peanuts, smoked salmon and oyster mushrooms, roast goose, cheese, port, champagne, Baileys and chocolates.

We had four more days before the fast, but while I got back on track, the photographer went totally off the detox rails. He consumed beer, Pringles, coffee and, as we waited for the Koh Samui connection at the airport, slipped in two Burger King chicken sandwiches, a huge pile of fried onion rings, a large Coke, followed by a chicken dinner on the plane. He was clearly heading for a remarkable first enema.

By the eve of the cleanse, I'd already lost over 2kg, weighing in at 86kg. Anthony was a little heavier, at 91kg. After demolishing an emotional last supper, we met our fellow fasters. They appeared a cosmopolitan crowd, confounding fears of being stranded among the sandals and lentil brigade.

There was Derek James, an engineer from Leeds, and Margaret Barrett, a sales rep from Cambridge, both in their mid-20s and aiming to clean up their acts after "caning it" while working in clubs in Tokyo. Nicky McCulloch, a 27-year-old Australian teacher, hoped to sort out a range of allergies, including wheat and alcohol. She was travelling with Mez Hay, a worm farmer with a shock of blond hair and strident ocker accent. Passionate about Italian food, along with steak, chops and sausages from her parents' farm, Mez admitted she was keeping her friend company and hadn't put in a single second's preparation. "I didn't know about it," she snapped. "Who the hell are you, the bloody fast police?"

Others also had tangible goals, including tackling stomach

complaints, severe constipation and mystery lumps. Most were keen to stress - a cynic might say too keen - that losing weight was not the goal. "It's a bit extreme to travel half way round the world just for a diet," argued Mez. "You'd be a bit superficial. Mind you, I wouldn't mind shedding a few pounds."

That didn't promise to be a problem. After checking our pH levels - too low and the fast isn't advisable - we immediately learned that while we wouldn't be eating, a great deal would still pass our lips. The relaxed, stress-free week on the beach would involve a Stalinist adherence to a pill-popping timetable. Each day started with a charming 7am detox cocktail of psyllium husk and bentonite clay. It had the texture of liquid cotton wool, but would be crucial for pushing toxins and garbage through my system.

Ninety minutes later, we had to swallow eight tablets. They looked like rabbit droppings, tasted like rabbit droppings but were, in fact, a mix of chompers (herbal laxatives and cleansers to attack the accumulated gunge in our colons) and herbal nutrients to help compensate for those missed during starvation. We had to repeat these two doses every three hours, every day, with a final handful of pills at 8.30 each night. There was just one more lesson, the small matter of the self-administered enema. Our teacher was the sickeningly lean, tanned resident alternative health expert, Chris Gaya, who appeared to have stepped straight out of a Californian aerobic video. He made the colonic irrigation equipment - bucket, piece of wood, plastic tube, bulldog clip and nozzle - sound like straightforward DIY, although it's unlikely to feature on Blue Peter in the near future.

All we had to do, he informed us, was to lie on the wooden board between a stool (stop giggling at the back) and the toilet basin. There's a hole at one end of the board over the loo; above it a nozzle connects to a tube, which in turn leads to a five-gallon bucket of liquid hanging from the ceiling. We would liberally coat the nozzle, which was the width of a Biro ink tube, with KY jelly, lie back, think of profiteroles with chocolate sauce, and slide on.

Controlling the flow of liquid with a bulldog clip, we were to let it flow until we felt full, before massaging it round the colon (roughly following three sides of a square around the lower belly) and releasing. Fluid would, apparently, be flowing in and out of our backside at the same time. "We'll be on the board for around 40 minutes," cooed Chris. "So let's make ourselves as relaxed as possible. Put on some soft music, light a candle, create a romantic atmosphere."

We clearly took different approaches to seduction. But mastering the enema, once I'd got over muscle-clenching nervousness, really wasn't difficult. I somehow ended up with my right foot half way up the wall, but five gallons went in and out without major trauma. By that night I'd shed another kilo, and although light-headed after 24 hours without food, felt strangely satisfied with the mix of supplements and detox drinks.

Next morning, my first enema of the day down the pan, I sat in the restaurant staring longingly at the menu, and found inspiration in the shape of two women nibbling their post-fast fruit. They exuded some of the rudest health I'd ever seen.

Carol Beauclerk, a "global nomad" with a mop of curly black hair, was a vegetarian, practised yoga, meditated and warmed up for her fast with a 17-day hike in Nepal. At 54, she had the energy and enthusiasm of someone half her age. "This place is really jumping," she enthused. "I'm now hoping to do a week-long fast each year."

Two tables away, scribbling in a diary, was Claire Lyons, a 32-year-old British journalist who had recently completed 21 days without eating. Having not gone near a set of scales, she had no idea how much weight she'd lost, but told me, "I feel great. Once I got past day 10, over the hump, it was surprisingly easy." Claire oozed serenity, but three weeks without food is unlikely to leave anyone hyperactive.

By mid-afternoon, their shining example was all but forgotten. I was feeling awful. Tired, lethargic, simply lousy. Having not eaten for 36 hours my body was apparently going into detox mode. Margaret, who had felt nauseous since waking, had actually thrown up, and was questioning her motivation. Nicky, meanwhile, had produced "something about nine inches long, it was very dark, very scary".

Things were no better for Mez. Already ravenous, she was spending an inordinate amount of time sniffing around plates of steaming Thai curry in the restaurant. She had also failed to grasp the basics of colonic irrigation. Instead of letting the liquid flow out, she had taken a massive amount in - until she was about to burst - before struggling to sit on the toilet and release it. "I had a huge stomach," she gasped. "I was thinking, this must be wrong. If anyone can take the whole bucket in one go, they're sensational." I made a mental note to watch out for spectacular explosions from chalet six.

It wasn't all bad news, however. I discovered we were allowed the luxury of a daily bowl of vegetable broth. It made me pathetically happy, savouring every drop as if it were a Gordon Ramsay creation. Filling perhaps, but it did little to halt the weight loss, and by the end of day two, a further two kilos had vanished.

By next morning, tiredness had been added to my hunger. I seemed to have been up half the night on the loo, the result of drinking a copious amount of fluid. My bodily functions had also taken a turn for the truly bizarre. I experienced flu-like symptoms as I started to expel 36 years' worth of toxins with headaches and aching muscles; my nose ran constantly, my eyes were sore and weepy, my ears waxy. I felt like something out of The Omen. I had also plucked up the nerve to put a colander down the toilet. Close examination showed I had passed several feet of long brown string that shimmered as if subtly illuminated by a photographer's light.

And I wasn't alone. Margaret had picked through her colander with chopsticks to reveal yellow fatty chunks, Mez had filled hers to the brim with brown stringy "chicken skin" mucus ("We're talking litres"), as had Derek, whose output included a strip about eight inches long, while Anthony described his as "patchy, like rabbit droppings". Similar surreal conversations with virtual strangers became the norm, achieving levels of intimacy beyond the range of couples who have been together for years. Perhaps avoiding frank discussion of bowel movements is one secret of a long-lasting relationship.

That night, as I escaped the dense tropical warmth, and flicked through books on diet and nutrition in The Spa's library, I discovered a remarkable document: The Healthview Newsletter. Inside, octogenarian bowel specialist, V E Irons, attempted the Herculean task of selling colonic irrigation on its erotic potential. I would lose my frigidity, he promised, my sex life would go stratospheric.

"How could anyone fully enjoy sex when he has up to 15 years of encrusted fecal matter and mucus in his colon?" asked Irons. "HE CAN'T - and HE WON'T. If you want to remain sexually potent for your entire life, start cleaning your colon today. I'm 87, and I still enjoy sex. And if I can at my age, I know you can at your age... so get on with it!" It was of little consolation to Mez, whose hunger had now assumed epic proportions. She was considering eating her apricot moisturiser, she told me.

That night produced the most vivid dreams of my life, a typical symptom of detox, with blockages disappearing from the mind as well as the body: I'd attacked Vietcong gun positions in a hot air balloon, I'd played golf with exploding balls, I'd been savaged by a grizzly bear. Other guests' dreams were more grounded in reality: Anthony and Mez had raided their parents' fridges, with the worm farmer devouring steak, potatoes and cheese sauce.

And some simply begged for the psychiatrist's couch. Nicky, who in reality sees her divorced father only sporadically, dreamed he had turned into her boyfriend. Freud would have enjoyed that. Indeed, in private conversations with guests, well away from my notebook, many fasters admitted to having recently split up, or having travelled to Koh Samui to get a long-distance perspective on relationships. I had unwittingly stumbled on Relate-On-Sea.

There was further physical fall-out, too. Day four was supposedly the worst of the week, with toxins expelled through the skin and lungs, as well as the kidney and colon. I didn't disappoint. My nose, ears and eyes deteriorated, my sinuses throbbed, I was yet more sluggish. It felt like a beer, wine and whisky hangover. Increasingly strange things appeared in our colanders. Derek was shocked to find rubbery nuggets, Mez had found black oval shapes "up to five inches long", my offering had an almost luminous green tint.

As if to celebrate crossing the halfway point of the week, many of us switched enema solutions. Abandoning coffee and vinegar, I flamboyantly opted for garlic, claimed to get rid of parasites. It seemed as natural as ordering gin and tonic instead of margarita, but when I casually told my girlfriend in a telephone call to London, there was a long silence. "Are you aware how tenuous your grip is on reality?" she asked. "Are you with a cult?"

I clearly needed to get out more. Many people hadn't left The Spa for days, it was developing its own micro-culture. But when I summoned up the energy to sip mineral water in a bar in nearby Lamai town, I felt instant paranoia. The lights, the noise, the crowds, the smell of food. It was a world in which I didn't belong.

I returned to the womb to find new guests. John Twigg, a burly 37-year-old Kiwi, had prepared by drinking more wine. "It's made of grapes," he argued. "Grapes are vegetables, so what's the problem?" He was joined by the Lycra-clad Mimi and Dave Hatherley from Fairbanks, Alaska, who had an unnerving habit of finishing each other's sentences. Forty-two-year-old Mimi ran, biked and did step classes five times a week; Dave, 43, ran, skied, hiked, climbed and mountain biked. They were both "into vitamins and nutrition" and while fasting were also exercising hard because "the results will be better". After talking to them, I felt strangely giddy.

My mood and physical condition, however, were about to go through a dramatic change. By lunch - sorry, by the second dose of herbal laxatives - on day five, my nose, eyes and ears had cleared, and I had more energy. Remarkably, without nibbling a single shred of food for 120 hours, the irrigation still washed out huge amounts of gunk. I passed six-inch strips of gristle and what appeared to be large chunks of fillet steak. I don't know how I ever afforded them, let alone swallowed them.

At least I could contribute to the increasingly competitive enema discussions. Someone had always passed something harder, brighter, more bizarre. Margaret's chopsticks had unearthed some gristle, about a foot long, and hard, black pellets. She was so impressed she took a photograph. A few chalets away, Mez had passed "rubbery brown, fat worms" with a strange purple glaze, which she insisted on showing to me in her bathroom. But the clear winner was Anthony's 22-year-old marble. Perhaps the most bizarre thing, which I didn't appreciate until days later, is that it all seemed perfectly normal at the time.

When I next bumped into Alaska Dave, he was jogging rapidly between the restaurant and his chalet. As panpipe music played in the background and he told me about today's three-mile hike, I noticed he wore a strange electrical device. It was a zapper that emitted an electrical current to kill parasites, and carried the printed warning: "For research only. Not approved for use on humans." Even for The Spa, that clearly wasn't normal.

The improvement continued into day six. A nearly detoxified brain and bloodstream meant I awoke clear-headed, and full of energy. The enemas now produced less, but it was darker and harder as the fast broke away the older, more ingrained plaque.

It was the same story the next day. Our bodies seemed to reflect a mood of demob happiness. I had rarely felt so healthy, so energised, in my adult life. That didn't, however, mean the end of the bizarre revelations. John passed "something from an alien movie" into his colander - and then videoed it for his office colleagues. He was joined by an outsized oil worker, Pipeline Pete, embarking on his 10th fast. "The first time I came," he boasted, "they needed to dig three cesspits."

And there were more. Early that evening, I found Mez huddled over a well-thumbed tome in the library. "Jesus, have you read some of these?" she groaned, handing me a book of ex-guests' awed testaments. "I'd have bet £1,000 my bowels were clean," wrote Chris Markvert, 67, "seldom have I been so surprised." "Great pooing," said Roy from San Francisco, "the best month of my young life." And RTM contributed seven pages of increasingly manic scrawl, which included interesting facts about the Vikings.

It also contained graphic photographs of people's enemas, footnotes in The Spa's history to go alongside stories of legendary guests, such as the alcoholic whose detox included hiding whisky bottles and wandering naked into neighbouring resorts; and "Kathmandu Joan", who fasted for 140 days over two and a half years, passing over 70 green and black "buttons" and clearing up an abdominal disorder.

We couldn't compete with that, but by the morning of day eight, the fast was being credited with impressive results. It had, people claimed, got rid of allergies; removed worrying lumps that had necessitated appointments with gynaecologists; eased severe period pains and sinus problems; helped people lose kilograms while improving their skin and strengthening their nails. I'd lost well over 6kg, had an indecent amount of energy and, as people kept observing, had developed unnaturally bright eyes. I wasn't aware they were cloudy before, but felt I had earned some flattery after 14 enemas and no food for roughly 170 hours, 35 minutes and four seconds. The cost of the seven-day programme, by the way, (was £184), and accommodation in a chalet for the week adds another £60 or so.

The first post-fast meal of papaya made my toes curl with pleasure, but, as George Bernard Shaw observed, "Any fool can fast, but it takes a wise man to break a fast properly." Raw fruit and vegetables should be the order of the next three days, but within hours Anthony had consumed two Snickers bars and a fish supper. It appeared to have no ill effects. They came 24 hours later. After demolishing piles of local prawns, we unwisely sipped a shot of Mekong whisky. Toxins tasted good, very good indeed. So good in fact, that by midnight, we had drunk a bottle each. The next morning, on the beach, my glasses were smashed, toxins pulsing around my bloodstream, the hangover indescribable.

But the week was not wasted. As a nutritional Philistine, I was inspired to read more, to learn some basic lessons. It's hardly double-blind scientific research, but I defy anyone to examine a post-irrigation colander with its chunks of apparently undigested family roast and not make some small changes to their diet. I love meat; the smell, the taste, the texture, but now it only makes a rare appearance on my plate.

Frankly, even that's too much for the gurus of cleansing, who believe a truly health diet revolves around fruit, vegetables, nuts and pulses - the more that's raw or steamed the better. Along with fish, they've become the staples of my diet. If I occasionally lapse - and nothing will make me give up Christmas turkey or goose - a flashback to The Spa reins me in.

While I'll take caffeine, alcohol and chocolate to the grave, I've also cut back on most dairy and wheat products. It might make me the dining companion from hell, but I do, at least, have the stories. People are constantly appalled yet fascinated by the idea of cleansing, and for some masochistic reason, demand the grim details between starter and main course. As they wait for their medium rare fillet or pork Dijonnaise, they crane forward to hear more about the decaying contents of people's colons.

As for Anthony, he never considered giving up meat. Or cream sauces. Certainly not Snickers. Life, as he sees it, is too short. And who am I to argue? But remember, this is the man who has lost his marble." Ian Belcher/ Guardian Newspapers

"Colonics: When the body has been under long-term attack by drugs (Yes, aspirin and alcohol are both drugs!) Salt, heavy metals (including dental mercury) toxic chemicals, parasites, harmful microbes their toxins and circulating immune complexes (immune cells locked onto undigested particles or other foreign substances circulating in the bloodstream), it produces mucoid plaque to protect itself" Dr. Richard Anderson N.D. NMD

Dr. Anderson is the guru of the *"Detox Movement"*. He

points out that once mucoid plaque has been created, for whatever reason, it is not routinely excreted from the large intestine. It lodges in the folds and crevices of the colon and can remain stuck there for many years. It slows down intestinal action in two ways. It brakes the excretory function and it prevents proper nutrient absorption. It provides a fertile breeding ground for pathogens and parasites and can block the outflow of lymph and mucin drainage. Evidently, this contributes to bowel toxicity; as toxins slowly build up they have a tendency to overflow into the bloodstream. This provides a perfect environment for the creation of *"dis-ease"* of all sorts including the formation of cancer. You need to clean the gut. What are you going to do about it?

Find somewhere that offers *"colonic irrigation"* treatment and sign up for a course. There are three types. 1) The *"Colema"* variety which is colorfully described in Ian Belcher's *"Guardian"* article.

2) The Open System. This is a more clinical variant of the *"Colema"*. Modern versions include beds, discreet tubes, and reverse osmosis water, in a process which is generally administered by a nurse or some other health care professional. The system is not pressurized, water flows according to the laws of gravity. The water includes additives like *"coffee"* that spurs the liver to let go toxins, *"Apple Cider Vinegar"* to alkalize the colon, making it a less attractive habitat for pathogens and parasites, and *"probiotics"* to replace the friendly gut bacteria that the colonic washes away. There are establishments located all over the world, similar to *"The Spa* "in Koh Samui that specialize in cleansing and fasting programs. Contact Health Ambit Consultancy and we can help you find a suitable venue in a region of the world that is convenient for you. Shame, though, you could come here to lovely Koh Samui in order to complete your detox!

healthambitconsultancy@protonmail.com

3) The Closed System: This differs from the "open variety"

based on gravity feed, because it's pressurized. The operator controls the treatment by allowing water to enter the colon, holding the liquid and then releasing it. In the open system, it is the client who decides when to "push out and release" the load; this is not the case in the closed. Which system is preferable is very much up to the individual. Some say the pressurized *"closed system"* could cause a perforation of the bowel. Yes, there is a very slender possibility of this occurring. If you feel concerned by this, plump for the *"open system"* or even the *"colema board"*. Remember, the purpose of colonics is to clean the gut. They are not primarily for weight loss where many other factors need to be taken into consideration. A warning, colonics are contra-indicated for pregnant women, people who have very high blood pressure, suffer from an eating disorder, have a perforated intestine or have a very low BMI. All responsible operators have an intake form and will screen you before allowing you to embark on the procedure.

Constipation: This condition is pan-endemic, due "principally to poor life-style choices" which include inadequate diet, lack of exercise and excessive stress. The Miracle Mineral *"Magnesium"* more often than not comes to the rescue here. If you are constipated start by taking a Magnesium supplement. The dosage should be 500 mg twice per day. Colonics, too are helpful. They will remove accumulated fecal matter, but they won't address the root cause. Constipation causes toxicity, so it is always a priority that the condition ceases. To treat: 1) Add more fiber to the diet. Everybody needs at least 30gms daily. 2) Drink more quality water! 3) Increase fruits and vegetables in the daily diet. We all need at least 7 servings but 10 would be better. Remember, smoothies are an easy way of taking in this quantity. 4) A cup of freshly ground coffee in the morning often promotes bathroom visits. Be sure to exclude sugar and milk, though! 5) Often constipation stems from low bile production. *"Bone Broth"* would be helpful 6) Taking laxatives is not the answer. They treat the symptom but not the cause. 7) Take Vitamin C to bowel tolerance level.

To some people having somebody *"stick a tube up your*

bum!" is a gruesome prospect and best avoided. Something a little gentler would be *"the coffee enema"*.

"Enemas" have been used throughout history by various cultures as a means of clearing pathogens and other "debris" from the colon. There is evidence the ancient Egyptians were familiar with the practice as it's mentioned in the *"Dead Sea Scrolls"*. It was, however, Native North Americans tribes who came up with *"coffee enemas"* when they included green beans in the water to purify the liver. Enemas were believed to be a truly valuable health tool in the United States and elsewhere until the start of the twentieth century. I grew up on a tea estate in what is now Sri Lanka, and remember vividly how the *"dispenser"* who served as the Dr. would prescribe enemas for a host of different conditions and this was well into the 1950s. Treatments did change as the twentieth century, dawned. In the USA both the *"charitable"* Rockefeller and Carnegie *"Foundations"* decided that medicine should be more standardized; this gave rise to the 1910 *"Flexner Report"*. The report recommended *"Pharmaceutical Medicine"* be placed center stage in the healing arena. The findings were adopted; the Rockefeller family motives were not entirely altruistic, as many of the drugs that comprise modern western medicine are derived from the petroleum industry which was the bedrock upon which their fortune lay.

In 1971, Dr. Kellogg reported in *"The Journal of American Medicine"*, that in his years of medical practice more than 40,000 cases of gastrointestinal disease had improved significantly due to the simple treatment of improved nutrition, enemas and exercise. Let the numbers speak for themselves!

We have talked about the dangers of several toxins including fluoride and chlorine, but we have only said a little about processed foods. The enormous food processing industry depends on selling packaged products that can effortlessly provide nourishment in a busy age. Much of what is produced suits the manufacturer and not the consumer. Ingredients clog up the digestive tract and stick to the sides of the intestines. This mess putrefies and forms pockets in the colon's lining. To isolate the poisons and protect itself, the system makes a mucoid plaque that envelops the decaying waste. Over time the plaque solidifies, it becomes hard to budge whilst also providing an ideal breeding ground for parasites. A stodgy carbohydrate diet comprising bread, pasta, pizza, sticky sweet desserts and potatoes proceeds slowly through the digestive process; this adds to the poisonous load, so that toxins escape from the gut, into the bloodstream further contaminating the body. The tainted blood then makes its way to the liver for cleaning. The liver has to work overtime to clear up the disorder. It is stressed and overburdened; it cannot function optimally and the result is *"dis-ease"*.

That takes us back to the cleansing power of colonics and enemas. In this case, it's *"coffee enemas"*. This is the simplest variant and they have been found to improve energy levels, to ease bloating, improve mood and of course reduce toxic levels. Why? Because they provide an exit route for the noxious overload. They also achieve something truly remarkable; they prod the liver to produce *"glutathione."* *"Glutathione"* is the *"mother"* of all anti-oxidants and the body can make its own supply! If you can make it, use it! Sadly poor diet, pollution, toxins, medications and radiation all interfere with *"glutathione"* production. Dr. Mark Hyman says: *"In treating chronically ill patients with Functional Medicine for more than 10 years, I have found that glutathione deficiency is present in nearly all very ill patients."*

Glutathione is a simple molecule, comprised of three protein-building amino acids----cysteine, glycine and our friend glutamine-----. Its secret power is the *"Sulfur"* contained in the combination. *"Sulfur "*is a sticky substance and bad things adhere to it as flies do to fly-paper. These *"baddies"* include free radicals and heavy metals including mercury. Not only does your body make this amazing stuff, it can also recycle it. But there is a but; it can't recycle *"glutathione "*if the toxic load is too high! Back we go to the critical importance of *"A Cat Has Nine Lives And So Do You"*.

HOW TO DO A
COFFEE ENEMA

One method of detoxing the liver is coffee enemas. While many conventional doctors scoff at the idea of coffee enemas, they were included in the Merck Manual (the world's best-selling medical textbook) until the mid-1970s as a treatment for a variety of conditions.

Coffee enemas are used to improve energy levels, prevent bloating, improve mood, and reduce toxicity of the whole body by prompting liver cleansing and tissue repair. They also jumpstart the production of glutathione (the "master antioxidant") which is a powerful detoxifying agent.

DIRECTIONS:

 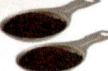 **Combine two tablespoons of organic, light roast ground coffee with 3 to 4 cups of filtered water.**

 **Bring coffee to a boil, simmer for 15 minutes and remove from heat.**

  Allow the coffee to cool (very important!)

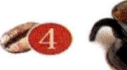 **Strain to remove any coffee grounds.**

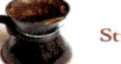 **Add to an enema pot or bag and administer as you would any enema. (Lie on your right side in fetal position with your knees bent inwards and up towards your stomach. Insert the nozzle about 2 inches into the rectum and allow the liquid to begin flowing.)**

   **Try and hold the liquid in for 10-15 minutes before releasing.**

Figure 8

58

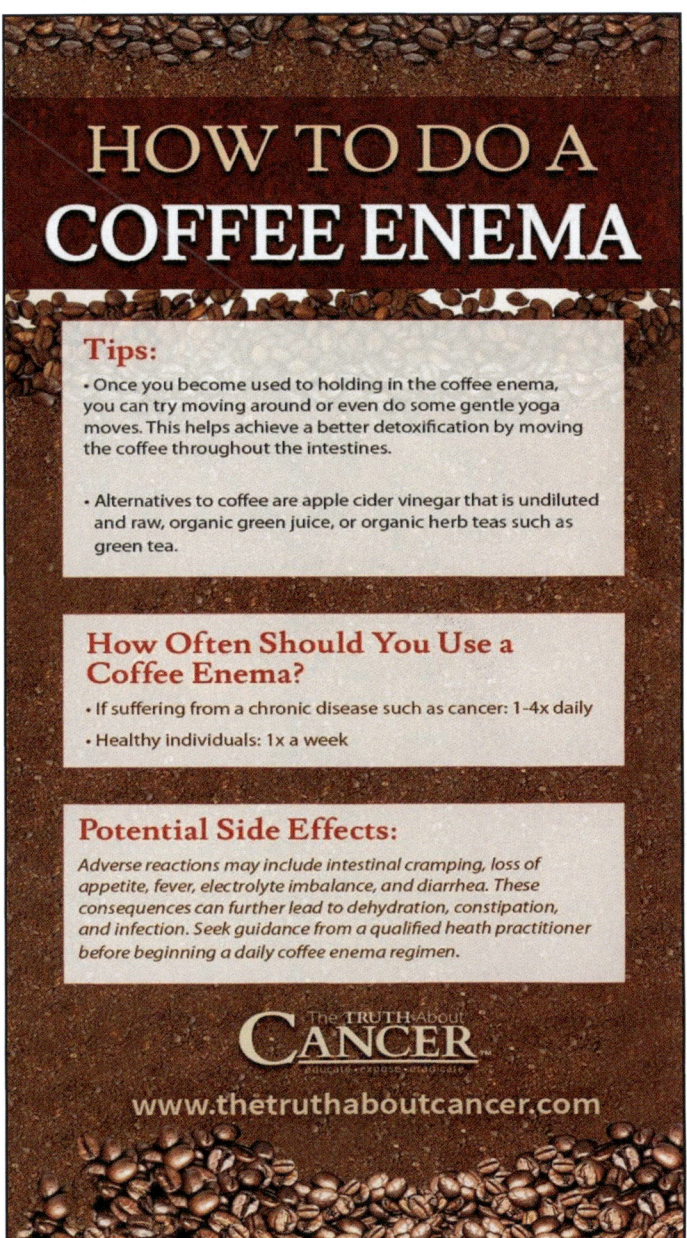

HOW TO DO A
COFFEE ENEMA

Tips:

• Once you become used to holding in the coffee enema, you can try moving around or even do some gentle yoga moves. This helps achieve a better detoxification by moving the coffee throughout the intestines.

• Alternatives to coffee are apple cider vinegar that is undiluted and raw, organic green juice, or organic herb teas such as green tea.

How Often Should You Use a Coffee Enema?

• If suffering from a chronic disease such as cancer: 1-4x daily

• Healthy individuals: 1x a week

Potential Side Effects:

Adverse reactions may include intestinal cramping, loss of appetite, fever, electrolyte imbalance, and diarrhea. These consequences can further lead to dehydration, constipation, and infection. Seek guidance from a qualified heath practitioner before beginning a daily coffee enema regimen.

The TRUTH About
CANCER
educate • expose • eradicate

www.thetruthaboutcancer.com

Studies have shown that green coffee beans boost "glutathione" by as much as 600% in the liver and an amazing 700% in the small intestine. Adding organic green coffee to colonics and enemas makes them very potent.

Dr. Max Gerson initiated *"The Gerson Therapy"* in the 1930s. The treatment protocol is still used in the treatment of cancer and other serious illnesses. The procedure is very strict. The diet mainly comprises living and uncooked vegetables, supplements and coffee enemas. The underlying notion is to remove toxins whilst simultaneously improving the efficiency of the immune system.

Gerson believed modern eating practices maintain an imbalance of Sodium and Potassium. We ingest too much Sodium and not enough Potassium. This includes potassium iodide, a crucial player in thyroid health. The imbalance is due mainly to the use of artificial fertilizers in modern agriculture. Please buy *"organic produce"* whenever possible.

OK, you've cleaned the gut------" THE MOTHER" of all organs---------Well done!

Of course none of the invasive *"colon cleansing techniques"*, might be your particular cup of tea. That's OK, too. We have another choice and that is the *"Herbal Detox"*. Here you take 5 supplement drinks per day for 8 days and eat salads and enzyme rich *"living foods",* enjoy juices and soups and experience a generally efficient *"clear out"*. Naturally, we would be delighted if you came to visit us here in Samui, but we can send you the herbs to make the *"drinks"*, give you instructions on what to eat and what juices to make and guide you through the *"Program"* via Skype, Line or What's App. If you would like to know more about this option, be sure to get in contact:

healthambitconsultancy@protonmail.com

Did you know the gut contains approximately 2 Kilos of bacteria? Some of this is good and some of it is bad. Ideally, 80% of this is lactic acid based *good stuff* "and the remainder is bad. Most of this inhabits the large intestine; 60% of stool is bacteria.

These friendly microorganisms are invaluable. They ferment unused *"energy resources"*; meaning glucose and the many glucose substitutes like fructose, maltose and some fatty acids which strain the immune system as end products of metabolism. *"Gut Flora"* prevents the growth of harmful species, so it is really part of the immune system. Yes, 60% of immunity lives in the colon and small intestine. The system also regulates the production of *"biotin" (B7)*, B12 and *"vitamin K"*. More than that, it makes hormones that aid in fat storage. Gut ecology is a vital force. It's destroyed by antibiotics; also by colonics and enemas! Gut cleansing sends toxins on their way but it also kills friendly bacteria. It's essential, therefore, after completing this second step in "A Cat Has Nine Lives And So Do You", that you work to restore the depleted *"good bacteria"*.

How Do We Do That?

To Reverse Possible Dysbacteriosis: Take Probiotics. As soon as your *"detox"* has finished start taking a good quality probiotic supplement. Initially, the dose is two capsules daily. Take them on an empty stomach, one probiotic first thing in the morning and the second last thing at night before bed. Stomach acid kills healthy bacteria; take the supplements when acid levels are at their lowest, and that is always away from food. Enteric coated varieties are available; some people insist the enteric coating protects the tiny living creatures from the high acid content of the stomach. According to *"The American Nutrition Association"*; most of the common probiotic organisms found in the *"Lactobacillus Bifidobacterium"* and *"Streptococcus"* species, like *"L. Acidophilus"* and *"L.Bifidus"* do not require enteric coating, because they can withstand the harsh stomach environment; if taken on an empty stomach, they will arrive at their requisite destinations in the small and large intestines largely intact. *"Lactobacillus Bulgaricus"*, however, and *"Streptococcus Thermophilus"*, will need an enteric protective coating.

"If I Eat Bio-Yogurt, Do I Still Need to Take Probiotics?"

The answer is probably *"yes"*. Most milk products are pasteurized by law. This is a heat processing treatment designed to kill the majority of bacteria. It does not matter if they are good or bad. Be very careful of the sugar laden commercial products like *"Yakult"*. These supposedly healthy yogurts contain more sugar than *"Coca-Cola"*. Their small, bottle-shaped containers are said by the company to contain live bacterial organisms. But I find it difficult to believe they can survive in such a sugar dense environment. Of course, sugar is essential in the fermentation process. Yeasts form and consume the sugars, but how can this be happening in a pre-packed yogurt that is refrigerated throughout the sales process? It beats me, so I suggest everybody steer well clear of these products. If you want a genuinely healthy probiotic strain that contains 42 different varieties of bacteria, let me suggest *"Bravo Probiotic Yogurt"*. It's made in Switzerland and comes in packs which you prepare yourself. It helps vital *"vitamin D"* assimilate and function correctly; beware though it is very expensive.

There are plenty of healthful foods available, containing lots of bacteria, which act very well as probiotics. Be sure to include one or more of them in your daily nutritional program. These fermented foods include Kimchi from Korea, Apple Cider Vinegar (use "Mother Tincture"), Sauerkraut, Kefir, cultured Coconut milk, Kombucha, fermented vegetables, Kvass, whey (not the protein whey usually made from Soya you buy in Health Food Stores) and at a pinch fermented Soya products like Miso and Natto (depends where they come from). Kvass is particularly delicious; it originates from the Ukraine and Russia and can be made from stale brown bread or beetroot. Bread Kvass is similar to non-alcoholic beer.

You Can Easily Ferment Vegetables and Make Your Own Probiotics.

Rejuvelac Cabbage Juice: Cabbage is an excellent vegetable to work with as its leaves are bacteria-rich so it ferments easily.

Finely chop up a head of cabbage.

Place it in a liter of spring water (Volvic is excellent)

Put the water in a large glass jar

Add the cabbage along with a clove of garlic.

Firmly close the jar

Leave to sit in an open space for three days

After three days, taste the mixture. If it is fizzy, it has fermented.

Place in the fridge to stop the fermentation and drink 30 ml twice daily.

How to Make Whey.

Buy a large container of natural plain yogurt.

Pour the yogurt into a cheesecloth or at least a thin cotton towel.

Suspend it above a bowl and allow the whey to drip through overnight. When the dripping stops pour the whey into a glass bottle and store in the fridge. Once refrigerated it will last for six months. You can use it to ferment vegetables, make salsas or even sauerkraut. The thick yogurt that still remains in the cheesecloth or thin towel is now cream cheese. Eat and enjoy! It's delicious when added to soups or salads.

Prebiotics: Prebiotics feed the probiotics. They are made of specific plant fibers, and they nourish the probiotics, now firmly ensconced in the large intestine. As far as we are concerned the fibers are indigestible but the more you have of them the happier your *"gut flora "*will be. How do you find them? Easy.....onions, garlic, raw wheat bran and bananas are the most common. The best prebiotic is raw "chicory root". It tastes similar to coffee. During World War 11, when it was difficult to ship coffee supplies to Europe they made a substitute made from chicory. In the UK they called it *"Camp Coffee"*. It came in bottles, looked like brown sauce and had a market well into the 1960s; it was disgusting! We all need fiber; most don't get enough! You won't get any in *"Camp Coffee"*, but you will from *"chicory root"*.

While we are on the subject of *"probiotics"*, it seems a good opportunity to re-introduce the subject of *"bone broth"*. Remember the healing powers of chicken soup as children. It or *"Brands Chicken Essence"* appeared at the onset of the merest sniffle. Some people affectionately referred to the soup as *"Jewish Penicillin"*. *"Bone Broth"* has similar properties and is used to treat a plethora of differing ailments.

Jordan Rubin is the founder of *"The Good Earth"* range of supplements. Products, incidentally I happily recommend. He tells of how Roman Gladiators did not eat T-Bone steaks and plump chicken breasts before fighting their bouts in the ring. No, these delicacies, by today's standards, were fed to the dogs. The Gladiators consumed the bones and cartilage of chickens, turkeys, beef and fish (does fish have cartilage?). These were slowly cooked up into huge soups which we now call *"bone broth"*. The slow cooking process breaks down the ingredients and is instrumental in building our own connective tissue by increasing reserves of gelatin collagen, loads of amino-acids along with a number of other nutrients including assimilatable potassium. This makes "bone broth" a super-food. It's easily digestible which marks it out as different from a number of other foods that irritate the digestive tract, causing discomfort and worst of all inflammation. Many avoid broth, believing it's hard to prepare, but with the correct equipment, it is really relatively easy. Firstly, you need a slow cooker. You will find the cookers easily and relatively cheaply in electrical outlets as well as certain supermarkets. Get hold of some bones and brown them in the oven (This step is very important). When browned take them out of the oven and place in the *"pot"* of your slow cooker, fill with spring water and add a selection of chopped vegetables. Onions, carrots, garlic, cabbage, tomatoes, spinach and broccoli are fine. To flavor include a generous pinch of sea salt, some black pepper as well as herbs like oregano, thyme and parsley. Turn on the slow cooker at a low setting and leave to bubble for the day. Dinner will be waiting for you, prepared and ready when you come home in the evening. Remove, the bones and drink the broth. You can add it to brown rice if you prefer a heavier dish, but it is better on its own.

The "Gaps Diet" (Gut and Psychology Syndrome) is a comprehensive protocol developed by Russian neurologist and nutritionist Dr. Natasha Campbell-McBride. The program evolved from *"The Special Carbohydrate Diet"*, created by Dr. Sidney Valentine Hass. The objective is evolving a way to naturally treat chronic inflammatory conditions in the digestive tract resulting from a damaged gut lining. Dr. Campbell-McBride developed her protocol to fit individual needs. She launched this rocket of discovery to heal her son who was born autistic. Her efforts were successful and she was happy to share her findings with others suffering from a variety of intestinal and neurological conditions. All these problems, she maintains, *"are due to an imbalanced bacterial "eco-system" within the G.I. tract"*.

The *"Gaps Diet"* focuses on removing foods that damage *"intestinal flora"* whilst replacing them with nutrition that *"heals and seals"* the gut. When the intestinal system has been repaired, then the offending items can be reintroduced slowly in keeping with the healing process. In line with the findings of *"A Cat Has Nine Lives And So Do You"*, we see *many* of our recommendations concur.

For instance, Dr. Campbell-McBride's diet restricts all grains, commercial dairy products, starchy vegetables and processed foods, particularly at the outset. Her focus is in keeping with the

"Bone Broth" formula, advocating homemade stock, stews and natural fats. Besides this, she recommends fermented foods and probiotics as well.

Simple Sensitivity Test:

If you feel you have a reaction to certain nutrients, there is a simple test that can be done at home. Take a drop of the suspect substance, if it is sold break it down into a paste with a little water. Place the drop on the inside of the wrist before going to bed. Go to sleep and check in the morning. If there is a red and angry reaction, you are sensitive. Cut the offending substance out of your diet. Test again when you have completed the *"Cat Has Nine Lives And So Do You"* Program. If then there is no reaction, you may re-introduce the food, but do so with caution and don't eat too much of it.

Life 3 – The Liver Cleanse

Time for the third step of *"A Cat Has Nine Lives And So Do You"*. We have cleaned the kidneys and the gut. Now we move to the largest organ of the lot, namely the liver. To be perfectly frank the liver is more of a gland than an organ. Why? Because a gland is a combination of tissue that excretes something. The liver excretes bile. Its principle function is to filter blood on its way from the digestive tract. Think of it as a factory designed to neutralize chemicals and other toxins. As it cleanses it also secretes bile; this emulsifies fats. The liver comprises a left and right lobe, whilst the gall-bladder sits underneath alongside parts of the pancreas and small intestine. The liver has a starring role in the digestive system.

Cholesterol is made in the liver. It has a special function and that is to transport fats. Glucose, too, is stored in the liver in the shape of glucagon. Iron lives here, too. As a result, it processes hemoglobin. It's iron that makes the blood red. Its presence in the center of every blood cell is its coloration factor. The end part of protein digestion is the formation of urea. It's a less toxic form of ammonia produced in the liver but filtered out into the urine via the kidney. As you can see the liver works very hard.

As a chemical filtration plant it can clog up with the poisons it's working to neutralize. These harmful substances are usually excreted into the bile for elimination via *"the poo"* whilst blood products are filtered out by the kidneys in *"the pee"*, but some can still end up sticking to the liver itself. That's why a liver *"detox"* is so important. If you have been abusing your liver through an excess of alcohol or drugs, ingesting a surfeit of sugar or enjoying a rich diet; then it's time for a liver *"rejuvenation"*.

Here's the test: mix some sea salt into a large glass of carbonated spring water (it **must** be carbonated). A half teaspoon of sea salt should give the water a salty *"tang"*. Squeeze the juice of half a fresh lemon into the mixture. This produces a zesty *"salty/lemon flavor"*. Drink slowly; the results are determined by the condition of your liver. If it's *"sick"*, you'll get loose bowels pretty quickly. This is not bad, but remember this! It's one of the principal routes the body rids itself of toxins. If the liver is ailing and "diarrhea" ensues, drink two glasses of the carbonated spring water and lemon/salt mixture every morning for a week. "Diarrhea" should stop as you go. Then you are ready to proceed to step 2. If nothing happened after the first glass, you can skip this step and go straight to the second one.

Liver Flush (5 Day Program)

Day 1. Take the juice of 1 lemon, one lime and half an orange. Place in blender with some spring water and ice. Add 1 tablespoon of extra virgin olive oil plus a small chunk of ginger and a slice of raw turmeric as well as 1 clove of garlic. Blend and drink

Day 2: Take the juice of 1 lemon, one lime and half an orange. Place in blender with some spring water and ice. Add 2 tablespoons of extra virgin olive oil plus a small chunk of ginger and a slice of raw turmeric as well as 2 cloves of garlic. Blend and drink.

Day 3: Take the juice of 1 lemon, one lime and half an orange. Place in blender with some spring water and ice. Add 3 tablespoons of extra virgin olive oil plus a small chunk of ginger and a slice of raw turmeric as well as 3 cloves of garlic. Blend and drink.

Day 4: Take the juice of 1 lemon, one lime and half an orange. Place in blender with some spring water and ice. Add 4 tablespoons of extra virgin olive oil plus a small chunk of ginger and a slice of raw turmeric as well as 4 cloves of garlic. Blend and drink.

Day 5: Take the juice of 1 lemon, one lime and half an orange. Place in blender with some spring water and ice. Add 5 tablespoons of extra virgin olive oil plus a small chunk of ginger and a slice of raw turmeric as well as 5 cloves of garlic. Blend and drink.

Take 4 "Propolis" tablet on each day of the cleanse. Propolis is a resinous substance that the bees take from buds and flowers to seal off spaces in the hive. This creates a healthier environment for their colony. Chinese researchers have found that this brownish substance incorporates"*isoferulic, sinapinic and caffeic acids"*. These are powerful antibacterial agents, which will kill-off the pathogens you release during the *"liver cleanse"*.

This is a semi-fast. Eat salads, soups and raw foods during the 5-day program. Drink lots of water, and use herbal teas. Avoid sugar and simple carbohydrates.

Eat Parsley to take away the garlic breath. Eat "living foods" Salads, Carrot Salads, Beet Salads, Gazpacho, Avocadoes, Potassium Broth Soup (this is cooked), Beet Juice, Wheatgrass juice. Drink, as well Green Juice that has been freshly made, and include smoothies, **only vegetables for the five days**.

When making smoothies with leafy green or cruciferous vegetables, it's recommended you cook them before use. Place in a pan, bring to the boil and then allow the water to cool off, remove vegetables and / place them in a blender. Brassica and other leafy greens should never be eaten raw as they contain lectins which are often toxic. Plants have their own defenses to keep predators at bay. Remember Canola Oil and its effect on cows? You don't want to suffer because of this.

Gallstones:

The renowned naturopath Hulda Clarke always proclaimed *"gallstones were produced in the liver;"* not in the gall-bladder as was popularly supposed. Gallstones form as a result of eating too many fried and fatty foods. That happens when these exceed the gall-bladder's capacity to break-down the fats. If you are flatulent after eating, then you have a clue your bile production is low and you need to take some steps to put the problem right. Excessive calcium and too many fats produce gallstones. The *"Liver Detox"* purges the system of the pesky stones. The olive oil opens the bile ducts, which allow the stones to make an easy exit. A precursor to the stones themselves is a silvery film made of the fat and calcium coagulating together. If you are having a problem with fat digestion, take *"granulated soya lecithin"* (this is one of the rare occasions I recommend soy products). Mix the grains with food; a tablespoon sprinkled on a salad or mixed in a smoothie will do the job. The protocol reduces blood fats and lipids. It is best to take two doses daily for a month and repeat bi-annually. You will find fat levels decreasing dramatically and digestion improving. Please use the granules and not the capsules, as their effect seems to be better. It's also wise to avoid deep-fried foods, fatty cheese and excessive amounts of butter. Always cook with Extra-Virgin Olive or Coconut Oil. Olive Oil begins to smoke at relatively low temperatures. This depends on the quality of the oil. Low-quality oil has a lower temperature *"smoke point."* You don't want it to burn as this will affect taste and cause the oil to oxidize. To overcome the problem, and this refers particularly to stir frying, start the process by frying the food with water. Cook with water over a high heat so it quickly evaporates, and then add the Olive Oil. At the moment there is a big controversy about the quality of many of the brands sold on the open market. Several are said to be of inferior quality. Olive Oil is light sensitive, meaning it should come in darkened bottles and needs to be *"greenish"* in color. Coconut Oil has a higher smoke point which makes it an easier cooking agent; it has, however, a strong flavor that many find unpleasant.

"Sugar spikes" show the liver to be overloaded; it's overworking to convert the glucose and store it as glycogen. When the process gets out of hand it has to change the sugars to fats before they damage the system. The crux of this matter is to find a way of controlling blood sugar. *"Chromium Picconolate"* provides an ideal solution. Another answer is *"chlorogenic acid"*, found mainly in green coffee beans. It has been touted by Dr. Oz and Oprah Winfrey as a miracle *"weight loss aid"*. Green coffee is bitter to drink and so not very nice. You will find a little *"chlorogenic acid"* in traditional roasted coffee. Coffee in this form has several health benefits. One of the most important is it promotes the flow of bile. This makes coffee is an Ideal after-meal drink for people with poor digestion. It also prevents sugar spikes and is an aid to blood sugar regulation. This excludes the enormous mugs served by the likes of *"Starbucks"*, which have the opposite effect!

Caffeine can disrupt sleep patterns so is not advisable after dinner or later in the day. However, coffee also contains anti-oxidants. There is a lot to be said for drinking quality coffee (instant coffee excluded) in smallish cups, a couple of times per day. There have been cases where it has been shown to reduce blood pressure, but quantity is the key. People used to have coffee services; the cups were thimble sized and were given to guests after the meal. That's how we should be drinking coffee. A cup in the morning, you may remember promotes bathroom visits, making it a pleasant constipation remedy. Beware though, coffee contains uric acid, a cause of gout. This acid quality causes dehydration and pH levels to drop, too. This is an instigator of acidosis. Acidosis creates a condition where alkaline bone calcium dissolves as this raises the dangerously low blood acid levels, but this, in turn, places too much calcium in the blood. If you consume an excess of fats, the calcium and fats amalgamate creating a plaque that then lines arteries; this is the mother of atherosclerosis. Like everything else small amounts of certain substances can promote good health but large quantities are harmful.

A word of caution directed at the ladies in particular. Firstly, women seem more prone to gallstones than men. The second factor that worsens the problem is rapid weight loss. When you shed weight too quickly the fat breakdown burdens both the liver and gallbladder which can cause gallstone formation. Weight loss programs are always best when they are slow and gentle as opposed to rapid and rigorous. Remember ,"BMIs" between 24-19 are the target. Athletes and bodybuilders will usually clock in with higher readings because muscle is heavier. Take your time to reach your goal. The end result will be much better.

Kidney-Bladder Cleanse Reminder

You began this three weeks ago under "*Life 1*". How are you doing? The "*detox*" is a great way to clean the urinary system. Hope your daily "*shots*" of parsley and coriander tea have paid off and you have experienced improvements. It's recommended you repeat this easy procedure before each "*liver cleanse*". Earlier I suggested you embark on two "*liver cleanses*" annually. Three weeks before your start, take a daily "*shot*" of the tea first thing every morning. Good cleansing to you!

Chaing Mai Study Shows Propolis Clears Up Cold Sores in a Matter of Hours.

"Bees are our helpers and our friends. It is estimated that 33% of human food production is dependent on insect pollination; most of this is accomplished by the honey bee. Sadly, the bee population is declining primarily due to the unconsidered use of petrochemical based pesticides and

chemicals. In some cases, beekeepers have been contracted to move their hives to areas devoid of bees to ensure pollination rather than to make honey.

Propolis is a resinous composition that bees collect from tree buds and certain flowers; it is used to seal off small spaces in the hive to protect it and improve the environment of the bee colony. Generally, brownish in color, it is proved by Chinese research to include isolated sinapinic, isoferulic and caffeic acids. These compounds have anti-bacterial properties. However, there is evidence too, that Propolis has anti-viral components.

A study conducted by Sirinad Musiaek and Yimanee Tragoolpua from the Biology Department at Chaing Mai University has revealed that Propolis extract, halted the Herpes Simplex Virus. Often associated with the common cold sore, Herpes Simplex 1 and 2 can affect various body areas namely the lips, eyes and skin. Transmission is often sexual; in the case of HSV 2, the genitals arc affected. It has been a causative factor in Cervical Cancer. The usual medical treatment is with the anti-viral drug Acyclovir. Many products flow from it; Zovirax is one of the best known. The treatment does not eliminate the cause, but it does address the symptoms. However, this can take up to four weeks in extreme cases and stress can easily trigger another outbreak. The remarkable Chiang Mai study showed that aqueous and ethanolic Propolis extracts altered the virus population on vitro cells after virus attachment in both Herpes Simplex 1 and 2 cases. Curiously the Propolis in high dosage performed better than Acyclovir in the case of HSV 2. The real test of the case lay in time, though. The study demonstrated how HSV-1 was entirely eliminated in a mere 60 minutes. It did, however, take just over 6 hours to remove the HSV-2 strain.

This is amazingly good news for the millions of Herpes sufferers worldwide, but there is even more to celebrate! That's because Acyclovir type drugs have been shown in rare cases to produce birth defects in neonates. A small US study of 467 pregnant women produced 17 birth defects in their off-spring. This shows a 3.6% affected rate, which is 0.6% higher than the *average birth defect rate of 3%. Is it worth taking a risk like this, however, slight? Women suffering from genital Herpes are expected to go on a course of Zovirax for the last few weeks of term to prevent lesions appearing at the time of birth. Wouldn't it be much better if they took safe Propolis instead during this crucial stage of fetal development? Secondly, it has been found that breast- feeding mothers pass on a large quantity of the anti-herpes medication to their babies whilst suckling. Again Propolis appears to solve the problem and no doubt benefits the infant, as well!*

Veerapan Tantipong is the President of Bee Products Industry Company Limited in Chaing Mai. He holds a BSc Degree from Chulalongkorn University in Bangkok. He has used his knowledge wisely and has come up with a solution for long-suffering Herpes victims. "Virulox", contains 50 mg of Propolis and a 120 mg of synergizing Royal Jelly in a lyophilized form. The tablet can pack a powerful punch of Propolis to help the sufferer overcome a Herpes attack. Take two tablets when you feel the first tingle of a cold sore and repeat the dose hourly for six hours. This alleviates the symptoms from both Herpes 1 and 2. The Propolis is aided by the 10 HDA in Royal Jelly, which some describe as being a precursor to the might of stem cells. But that's a story in itself!" **Alister Bredee**

Life 4 – Cleansing the Lymph

The lymphatic system is a network of tissues and organs that help rid the body of toxins. Its primary function is the transportation of lymph fluid. This colorless liquid contains white blood cells whose work comprise the destruction of infection.

The system contains the lymph vessels; they resemble the circulatory system but they lack the benefit of a central *"pump"*, namely the heart. These vessels are connected to nodes, located beneath the surface of the skin, clustering principally around key areas like the lungs and the heart. They rise close to the surface under the arms and in the groin. The largest *"lymphatic organ"* is the spleen. This is a major player in the immune system. It stores red blood cells and when it detects an invasion it flings out white cells or lymphocytes to ward off the attacking bacteria, virus or microorganism. This army of lymphocytes produces antibodies; a weapon designed to kill the foreign invader.

The tonsils, adenoids, spleen and thymus are all part of the lymphatic team. The thymus, located beneath the breast-bone, just above the heart, is where young lymphocytes are sent by their parents in bone marrow, to learn how to become mature and valuable *"T"* cells. The job of *"T"* cells is to go out and destroy infected or cancer cells. The thymus is very susceptible to stress. When overwhelmed it begins to shrink. It's important if you want a fully functioning immune system to keep the thymus in tip top shape.

Here's a simple little trick you can use to insure it works well. You tap it. Tap 7 or 8 times with an open palm from time to time throughout the day. This is particularly important after you have experienced a stressful event. According to Dr. John Diamond author of *"Life Energy: Unlocking the Hidden Power of Your Emotions to Achieve Total Well Being,"* the thymus regulates the energy flow of the body as well as the immune system and acts as a bridge between the body and the mind. A gentle tap sends it a small electrical charge that jump starts it to work better.

Lymph fluid is derived from blood plasma. Unlike the circulatory system of blood, lymph does not flow in a continuous loop but upwards towards the neck. The biggest problem with lymph is the enlargement of the nodes, which cause swelling. For the main part enlarged nodes are not dangerous; when they occur they show the body is combatting infection by siphoning off toxins and then cleaning them, but the result can be uncomfortable.

Manual Lymphatic Drainage is a type of Lymphatic Massage developed by Dr. Emil Vodder in the 1930s. It is now a familiar and much in demand physical therapy. This is a gentle touch technique during which the skin is stretched in a very precise direction. This prompts the lymph vessels to draw more fluid out of the tissue and into the lymphatic system for subsequent evacuation from the body. Think of it as a garbage collection service where protein molecules, water, dead cells and other detritus are swept away via the exit points located under the arms and in the groin. If you can find a therapist trained in this technique, I would urge you to go and seek some treatment. This is particularly important if you have fluid in the legs or feet. Whatever, you do, never underestimate the critical importance of movement. We all sit around far too much; this causes lymph to build up. Learn to move regularly. If you sit at a desk, get up and have a short walk around the office every hour. Don't sit still for long periods.

Any form of exercise that causes you to move up and down is really helpful. Skipping is one solution; it's an outstanding aerobic exercise and so is *"rebounding"*. A *"rebounder"* is a small trampoline. You can find them in *"Sports Equipment Stores"* as well as Amazon. Bouncing on these trampolines is a lot of fun and is definitely one of the best ways of getting lymphatic fluid to circulate. As it is three times more prevalent than blood there's a lot to shift around. Gently bouncing up and down on the *"rebounder"* creates increased *"G-Force"* resistance; this positively stresses every cell in the body. Lymphatic circulation is enhanced because the 1,000,000 tiny one-way valves are forced to function. It's important to remember that lymph always flows in one direction and that is towards the heart.

There are 3 Basic Rebounding Exercises:

1/ The Health Bounce. This involves gently bouncing up and down without your feet leaving the surface of the trampoline. This low impact exercise requires very little effort, but it efficiently moves lymph.

2/ The Strength Bounce is more vigorous. You jump as high as you can on and off the *"rebounder"*. It strengthens and stabilizes muscles, improves balance and really shakes up the lymph.

3/ Aerobic Bouncing. This one is for the experts. Use the *"rebounder"*to do jumping jacks, twisting, running in place and many more skilled maneuvers. These are high-density aerobic exercises reserved only for the fittest and most adept. This will definitely shake the lymphatic system into action, but please keep well away from these exercises if you are a beginner. You could hurt yourself; be careful!

The starting place for beginners is to sit on the mini-trampoline and gently bounce from a seated position. This is mild but it will still help the lymphatics. As you begin to feel more comfortable you can progress to more complex movements.

Neurolymphatic Reflexes

These are reflex points that stimulate the flow of lymph fluid. They are located all over the body, but the population is denser on the chest and the upper portion of the legs. When these points are massaged, toxins in the system are persuaded to move away rapidly. The points were discovered by Osteopath Frank Chapman in the 1930s. They are a mainstay of Kinesiology where the areas are known as *"lymphatic reflexes"*. It's useful to know the points because Donna Eden reassures us, they will:

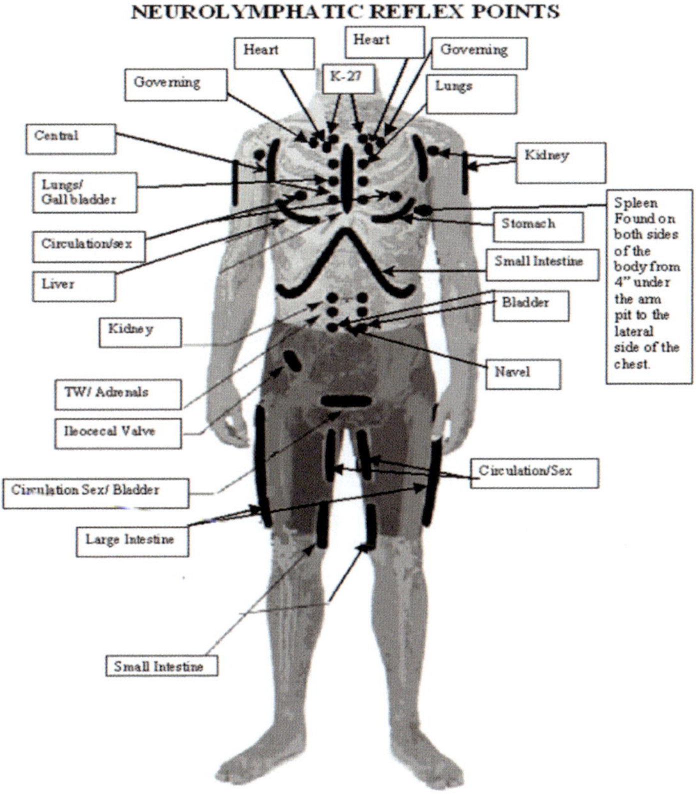

NEUROLYMPHATIC REFLEX POINTS

Figure 9

"Energize!
Send toxins to the lymphatic drainage system for removal
and clear away stagnant body energies; these include
emotional residue."

Skin Brushing

Here's a daily exercise to promote lymph flow.

Select a natural bristle brush (definitely not plastic). Needs to be relatively strong.

Brush rigorously upwards from the feet in the direction of

the heart.

When brushing the arms and upper body, always move towards the heart in keeping with the natural flow of lymph.

Now Let's Use the Reflexes

Look at the diagram above. Check out the points so it is easier to identify them. Gently massage each of them in turn. If you find a sore point, it needs work because it's congested. Massage until the tenderness reduces. Then move on to the next one. Warning! Don't massage too many at one time as you will release too many toxins all at once and this will overload the system. Don't be too rough, either, otherwise, you are likely to be black and blue with bruises. Work daily on the points with the aid of the diagram; over time you will notice the points become less sensitive because you have cleared them of toxins. Repeat this every three months to keep the lymphatic system in top shape.

The Lymphatic Massage

This one is fun. Teach your friend or partner how to give you a lymphatic massage. The map above shows *"the neurolymphatic reflexes"* on the front of the body; these points are easily accessible. However, major *"neurolymphatic reflexes"* affecting every meridian run either side of the spine. You can't reach them yourself, but you can easily get a friend to do it for you. This one comes from Donna Eden, too.

Lie face down or stand about a meter away from a wall, lean into the wall, supported by your hands. This allows your partner to work easily on your back.

Your partner then strongly massages the points along both sides of the spine, using the thumbs aided by body weight. Start at the neck area and work all the way to the tailbone.

Next, tell your friend to massage in the notches between each vertebra. Using the thumbs, lean into the point and stimulate each point for at least three seconds. Tell your partner to move the skin in a circular motion. Strong pressure is best, but not so strong the experience becomes uncomfortable.

When your massage partner reaches the sacrum, you can ask for a repeat or you can finish there. Tell your friend to *"sweep"* energy down your body from the shoulders. He/she does that with an open hand working down the body and legs and off the feet. This is best repeated two or three times. Rather than complicating the issue by inquiring which meridians are affected, simply ask for special attention on any sore spots that show up. The massage removes toxins from the lymphatic system, but it also stimulates cerebrospinal fluid. It is a tremendous immune system booster, too. If you feel the onset of a cold a *"neurolymphatic"* massage of this kind will usually stop it dead in its tracks! It also serves as a relationship *"bonder,* as it breaks down built up stress and tension which frequently pops to the surface during those difficult moments which often lead to arguments. Instead of fighting, get up against the wall and have your significant other give you a *"neurolymphatic"* massage.

If you have any subluxations or displaced vertebrae, you need to take action. It's stressful and displacements like these cause the body to go into stress related *"fight and flight"* mode. When you are in this state, hormones flood the system to prepare you to cope with emergencies. *"Cortisol "*increases and brings with it myriad problems. Yes, of course, you need to incorporate relaxation inducing tools like yoga and meditation into your life and include soothing foods which are high in vitamin B6. These are essential; they include sweet potatoes, pumpkin seeds along with seafood. High blood levels of B6 are crucial for immune system boosting which keeps *"dis-ease"* at bay. But you also need to see an osteopath or a chiropractor to straighten out any *"mis-alignments"* you may have.

Did you know that like teeth, vertebrae have a direct relationship to organs and can be the root cause of *"un-wellness?"* Let's take C1 (Cervical 1----The Atlas) A misalignment in this part of the neck causes serious issues ranging from head colds to high blood pressure, migraines, dizziness, chronic tiredness and even nervous breakdowns. If we move to T2 (Thoracic 2) we see a direct connection to the heart, its valves and the coronary arteries. It's odd to think a displaced T2 can be the cause of functional heart conditions and ongoing chest pain. It's always a good idea to have a check-up with a *"bodyworker"* like a chiropractor or osteopath, so problems can be straightened out and *"zestful fitness and good health"* become the order of the day. Just to bring this home loud and clear, here are some more examples. T8, for example, connects to the immune system. If your T8 needs adjustment, then you are likely to have ongoing low immunity which frequently shows up in colds and flu and other nagging health issues. L3 (Lumbar 3) connects to the sex organs as well as bladder, uterus, the knee, prostate and large intestine. If impotence is an issue, here is a good place to look. You can take Viagra until the cows come home, but you are simply wasting money. Interestingly, Viagra is one of the biggest selling pharmaceutical drugs on the planet and yet it has only a 38% efficiency rating, which in medical terms is considered good. Boldly speaking, it only works for 38% of its users. That means it is useless for 62% of the others. These spinal connections are not immediately obvious and will often be ignored by the medical profession, but they could often be a solution to an ongoing health issue which nobody seems to be able to resolve. It always pays to check these things out.

Get Lymphatic Fluid to Flow with the FAR Infrared Sauna

The spectrum of energy from the Sun is classified by the length of the emitted rays. The shortest are the most damaging and they are known as *"gamma rays"*. At the other end of the spectrum, but before the rays become *"radio"* waves, we come to the *"infrared"* band. If we move to the far end of that strata we arrive at the longest and most healing rays, this is the FAR Infrared range. The FAR infrared (FIR) frequency spans from 430 THz down to 300 GHz. It's these rays that bring about photosynthesis without which plants would not grow and life itself would come to an end on earth. Some people claim that healing modalities like *"Reiki"* comprise an energy similar to FAR Infrared.

The FIR system uses a zirconium, ceramic infrared heater emitting between 2 and 25 microns. These rays allow subcutaneous skin penetration of up to 4 cm. This type of sauna reduces lactic acid build up. Lactic acid increases after exercise; it is generally responsible for muscle pain. It stimulates endorphins (happy hormones) whilst killing bacteria and parasites. Its most important function, however, is to penetrate tissue, detoxify cells, inhibit swelling, improve lymph and blood circulatory flow and attract calcium to cell membranes where it can participate in healing. The key to the system is how the rays decrease the size of water clusters, allowing them better penetration both in and out of body tissue. This eases release of previously stuck toxins. The Sauna is a great way of clearing pesticides and herbicides which are usually surrendered through the urine, the stool and sweat. Colonics and enemas eliminate toxins via the bowel but Mayo Clinic studies have shown the FIR Sauna System to be a highly effective means of *"detoxing"* via the skin, and one of the safest ways when it comes to those with heart disease and blood pressure issues. The manufacturers of the Sauna boldly claim that a half hour session will help get rid of subcutaneous fat and burn up to 600 calories. This compares to 330 calories in half an hour's jogging! Saunas like this are excellent *"detox"* tools. Do try them if you get the opportunity. However, please avoid, if you are pregnant or have a pacemaker or stents. The experience will make you sweat buckets, so be very sure you are well hydrated before and during the process.

The Ileo-Cecal Valve

The Ileo-Cecal valve is a small muscle located on the right side between the large and small intestine. This one-way check valve allows food to pass from the small to the large intestine for further processing. Its proper function is to open and close on demand. It can stick in the open position, this causes a back-wash into the small intestine, which allows fecal matter to enter the blood. This has harmful effects in the small intestine where the fueling that ultimately feeds us, takes place. When this little muscle sticks in the closed position, waste cannot flow out into the bowel for elimination. Either the sticking open or the closing of the Ileo-Cecal create toxic conditions which can cause problems anywhere that blood flows.

Ileo-Cecal problems occur due to poor diet and emotional stress, both of which can seriously affect overall health. You can frequently identify a person with an Ileo-Cecal problem because they have a *"whining"* timbre to the voice. The liver meridian travels directly over this valve. High alcohol intake will stress it, causing it to stick open. This is a major factor in hangovers. People with ICV problems are:

Often grumpy
Have frequent mood changes
Are cranky
Are contrary
Are frequently tired
Have low energy
Have dark circles under the eyes (indication of toxicity)
Drag their feet
Suffer from cramps
Feel hot
Express a temper
Have headaches
Often get *"flu"*.
Have an attitude
When the valve is stuck in the open position:
Often suffer from flu and the common cold

Have frequent bowel movements

Experience muscle aches

Get recurring fevers (this is the body's attempt to cleanse itself by using heat to force toxins out via the skin in the form of sweat)

Have foggy thinking

Experience blurred vision

Have difficulty assimilating information

When the valve is stuck in the closed position:

Have elimination difficulties

Experience constipation

Can be the root cause of appendicitis (appendix becomes inflamed in its effort to neutralize toxins. The appendix is part of the lymph system)

Find it difficult to let go

Experience over-attachment to situations, people and conditions

If three or more of these symptoms persist, it is possible you have an Ileo-Cecal valve issue. Correct it and see if the symptoms disappear. You will have to repeat the correction over a ten day period in order to experience the improvement. A one off, won't do it!

Correction Technique

Use the same procedure to correct an open or a closed valve.

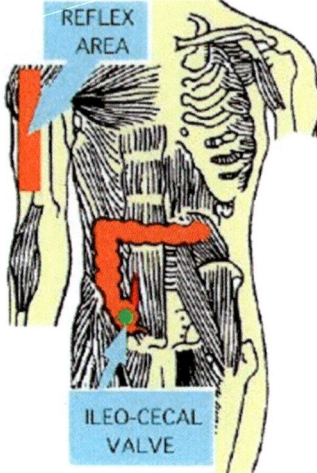

Figure 10

At the area of the valve (in two inches and down two inches from the top of the right hip). Massage with medium pressure in a clockwise circular motion for five seconds. Then using a closed fist, briskly stimulate the reflex area as indicated on the upper right arm for ten seconds.

Perform the correction daily for the minimum of ten days,

What to Expect When the Valve is Functioning Correctly

You will feel more connected to people, places and events

- You will feel more positive
- Have more energy
- Feel happier
- Sleep better

- Have regular bowel movements
- Eliminate muscle aches
- Experience more complete digestion
- Have clearer vision
- Enjoy more smiles

Now isn't that reason enough to try this simple little exercise?

Life 5 – The Parasite Cleanse

The late Dr. Hulda Clarke says when it comes to disease there are only two factors to consider........*pollutants and parasites*.

Flatworms, roundworms, protozoa and pinworms are all easy to destroy. It's the eggs and the larvae that pose the problem!

This is what to do. Take Black Walnut Hull Tincture (extra strength). It was the native North Americans who first used black walnut hulls as a laxative and then came to realize they eliminated parasites as well. This is because toxic *"juglone"* is found in black walnut, and this kills the parasites. It's effective against pinworms, ringworm, tapeworms and several insects and other assorted intestinal parasites. At the same time as the *"black walnut"* take *"wormwood"* capsules. Wormwood is the key ingredient in the drink *"absinthe"*, beloved elixir of the Parisian Bohemian set and popularized by the artist Toulouse Lautrec. Medieval sources record it served as a useful insecticide. It possesses a volatile oil, a cocktail within itself, containing essential oils theorine, cadinene, phellandrone and pinene. No wonder drinking *"absinthe"* was said to be a powerful hallucinogenic that would make you blind. *"The Green*

Fairy "as it was called, had such a bad reputation that it was banned in many countries including France and Switzerland in the early 1900s. The essential oils dispel parasites, particularly roundworms. Take too large a dose and you'll get diarrhea; it stimulates the emptying of the intestines. It is also a useful digestive aid as the bitter taste prompts the gallbladder to make bile.

Killing the parasites is easy, but the eggs and larvae are a different story. For instance, the *"enteriobus vermicularis"* (human pinworm) is the most common intestinal parasite in Europe and the USA. The worms live in the small intestine, but the gravid female travels to the anus to lay her eggs, usually in the middle of the night. The hatched larvae will then make their way back into the large intestine where they cause more infection. This process causes embarrassing anal itching, which is a giveaway sign that something is wrong.

Not all parasite eggs hatch in the body. For example, the common roundworm (Ascaris Lumbricoides), is the most prevalent species from a worldwide point of view. The adult female lays her eggs in the intestines of the infected person. The eggs exit via the feces; they can live in the soil for up to two years; when people eat vegetables or drink water that comes from the contaminated ground, they swallow the eggs and become infected themselves. The larvae then travel to the lungs and throat where they are swallowed, so arriving back in the intestines to start the process all over again.

It's Imperative You Wash Your Fruit and Vegetables

Wash produce thoroughly, simply rinsing under the tap will not suffice. Soak in a dilute solution of hydrogen peroxide (minimum 3% strength) for twenty minutes, this should kill parasites and their larvae. Eggs can appear in contaminated tap water, which is a very good reason never to drink it. Flukes, parasites and eggs can also appear in undercooked meat. Always make sure it is cooked properly, especially pork.

Cloves Kill Eggs

You need to make a *"tincture of cloves"* solution. Pour a bottle of vodka or some other white spirit into a plastic bowl or bucket. Cheap spirits like this are easily available; for the sake of your liver they are best, not drunk! Add a large packet of cloves. You will find them in most supermarkets. Allow the cloves to thoroughly soak in the alcohol. The liquid will turn black in a few days. Be very cautious when handling as it stains. Bottle the liquid and keep in a warm, dark place.

The Parasite Cleanse

This program spans the two week period between the New Moon and the Full Moon. Parasites move and become more active during this time. The program is repeated from New Moon to Full Moon for three consecutive months.

Day 1. Take 1 drop of Black Walnut tincture in water on an empty stomach, plus 1 drop of tincture of cloves. Take 1X 200mg capsule of wormwood before supper.

Day 2. Take 2 drops of Black Walnut tincture in water on an empty stomach, plus 2 drops of tincture of cloves. Take 1X 200mg capsule of wormwood before supper.

Day 3. Take 3 drops of Black Walnut tincture in water on an empty stomach, plus 3 drops of tincture of cloves. Take 2X 200mg capsules of wormwood before supper.

Day 4. Take 4 drops of Black Walnut tincture in water on an empty stomach, plus 4 drops of tincture of cloves. Take 2X 200mg capsules of wormwood before supper.

Day 5. Take 5 drops of Black Walnut tincture in water on an empty stomach, plus 5 drops of tincture of cloves. Take 3X 200mg capsules of wormwood before supper.

Day 6. Take 6 drops of Black Walnut tincture in water on an empty stomach, plus 6 drops of tincture of cloves. Take 3X 200mg capsules of wormwood before supper.

Day 7. Take 7 drops of Black Walnut tincture in water on an empty stomach, plus 7 drops of tincture of cloves. Take 4X 200mg capsules of wormwood before supper.

Day 8. Take 8 drops of Black Walnut tincture in water on an empty stomach, plus 8 drops of tincture of cloves. Take 4X 200mg capsules of wormwood before supper.

Day 9. Take 9 drops of Black Walnut tincture in water on an empty stomach, plus 9 drops of tincture of cloves. Take 4X 200mg capsules of wormwood before supper.

Day 10. Take 10 drops of Black Walnut tincture in water on an empty stomach, plus 10 drops of tincture of cloves. Take 5X 200mg capsules of wormwood before supper.

Day 11. Take 11 drops of Black Walnut tincture in water on an empty stomach, plus 11 drops of tincture of cloves. Take 5X 200mg capsules of wormwood before supper.

Day 12. Take 12 drops of Black Walnut tincture in water on an empty stomach, plus 12 drops of tincture of cloves. Take 6X 200mg capsules of wormwood before supper.

Day 13. Take 13 drops of Black Walnut tincture in water on an empty stomach, plus 13 drops of tincture of cloves. Take 6X 200mg capsules of wormwood before supper.

Day 14. Take 14 drops of Black Walnut tincture in water on an empty stomach, plus 14 drops of tincture of cloves. Take 7X 200mg capsules of wormwood before supper.

*Note the larger doses of wormwood, could result in loose stools. This is good, as it will expel the parasites more quickly. If you find it uncomfortable cut back the dosage

Finish and repeat over the next consecutive two months. Repeat the *"detox"* every year.

Pets

We all love our pets very dearly, but as they spend a lot of time snuffling and rooting around on the ground, they pick up parasites very easily. Be sure to go to your vet and get worming tablets for them. You need to do this every six months, otherwise, they will be reinfecting you.

Getting the Products

There are several websites selling these products. In the USA, I recommend Kroeger Herb.

www.kroegerherb.com

The Organic Nutrition Company is based in both the UK and the USA. Their UK base is in West Sussex.

https://www.organicnutrition.co.uk/proof.htm

Some Other Tips

Ascorbic acid is a wonderful parasite killer. Look out for the powdered or crystalline form. Add a small spoon to your smoothies and juices. This will be sure to polish off anything that might have survived your cleaning process. A small spoonful equals about 5 Gms. Another trick is grain alcohol. Vodka or white spirits will do fine. Keep a handy supply in a spray bottle. You can squirt this onto foods after cleaning and before cooking in order to be very sure. It also serves as a handy bathroom spray. Vodka will kill parasites and larvae that might get on your hands. This is particularly useful with pets and young children, especially when they have" *bathroom accidents"*. Be sure to clean toilet surfaces with the vodka as well as chopping boards and kitchen surfaces that come into contact with food. Note: Don't drink the vodka. It's cleaning fluid!

Low Stomach Acid Makes Parasite Infection Easier:

To check to see whether you have adequate levels of stomach acid, try this simple test.

Put a quarter teaspoon of bicarbonate of soda in an 8 oz. (240 ml) glass of water. Drink this first thing one morning.

Time how long it takes to *"belch"*. If you produce adequate stomach acid you will within 2/3 minutes.

Early and repeated *"belching"* is a sign of excessive stomach acid (rare!). If you do not respond or it takes a long time to *"belch"*, you have low levels. The *"belch"* results from acid and base (Sodium Bicarbonate) reacting to form CO_2.

If you have low stomach acid, you might have a gut full of *"ascaris"*. Try a parasite cleanse and see if there is a difference. Can it get any simpler than that?

Dr. Simon Yu, writing in his book *"Accidental Cures"* tells of a Medical Mission to Bolivia that first introduced him to the hidden dangers of parasites:

"Since my first-hand experience in Bolivia, I've used parasite medications in various combinations. I've observed dramatic responses in my patients in situations where specialists' treatments had failed. Some of the difficult conditions that responded with parasite medications included: intractable allergies and asthma, migraine headache, sciatica, constipation and diarrhea, irritable bowel syndrome, colitis, bronchiectasis, vision loss, anxiety, depression, nightmares, TMJ (temporomandibular joint) problems, chronic fatigue, fibromyalgia, multiple sclerosis, arthralgia and myalgia, pelvic pain, eczema, psoriasis, hypertension, and others."

Life 6 – Cleansing the Heavy Metals

Today the FDA in the USA tell pregnant women to limit their intake of tuna fish to 6 ozs per week. That equals 70 Gms, not very much! Why? The warning is in effect because it seems tuna contains mercury, and this can harm the developing fetus. If you feel unsure about heavy metals in your system, you can have a blood test which will show up mercury, lead, cadmium and arsenic levels. The accuracy of the test is suspect because the heavy metals accumulate in the organs and not in the blood. Lead toxicity is extremely common. It was used extensively in high-octane gasoline, which happily has now been phased out. Lead, though still appears in some old water piping. One of its effects is to reduce IQ. One could say it dumbs people down! Mercury is definitely another huge problem. Dr. Simon Yu in *"Accidental Cures"* warns that a combination of lead and mercury create what he calls *"synergistic toxic effects"*. This means that combined together the presence of both metals increases the overall toxic effect an amazing one hundredfold.

Mercury is considered to be the most toxic substance on earth that is if you exclude the radioactive elements like plutonium. In spite of this dentists still insist that mercury is safe and continue to use amalgams to fill teeth, whilst Thimerosal is found as a preservative in some vaccines. Thimerosal contains 49.5% mercury; it is certainly included to counteract mold in the Flu vaccine. Who would want this potent *"neuro-immune"* toxin injected into themselves anyway? It seems you can request a *"mercury free"* variant, but you have to understand the situation before you can make the appeal. On September 11th, 2014, ever popular TV presenter Dr. Oz stated that Thimerosal had been removed from all childhood vaccines. According to Vax Truth, this is not necessarily true.

"The FDA changed the rules so vaccine manufacturers do not have to include Thimerosal on the label as an ingredient unless it is used as a preservative. According to the FDA, if Thimerosal is used in the manufacturing process but it is not used as a preservative, the vaccine can be labelled "Thimerosal-free" when that is not the case The point is, several vaccines given to infants and children still contain Thimerosal, including the DTaP vaccine, DT vaccine, Hib (ACTHib, TriHIBit) and Meningococcal vaccine.....the meningococcal vaccine given to children age two years and older contains the same amount of Thimerosal (50 mcg.) as the multi-dose flu shots." Vax Truth:

http://www.vaxtruth.org/2014/09/Dr-oz.-flu-shots/

Something Dr. Oz failed to mention was aluminum, which is present in a whole slew of vaccines. It is toxic and like mercury constitutes a powerful *"neuro-immune"* poison. Everybody is focusing on mercury whilst even more harmful aluminum is slipping under the radar. Apoptosis is when cells die off naturally and are then replaced by new cells. Aluminum accrues to toxic levels especially in those cells like the bones, the heart and the brain, where apoptosis is slow. The brain and the associated nervous system are where diseases like Alzheimer's, Parkinson's, Multiple Sclerosis, Chronic Fatigue and neurological or auto-immune problems manifest. This includes the complete autistic spectrum, including ADD and ADHD as well as full blown autism. The number of children diagnosed as autistic has grown alarmingly over the years. In the 1970s approximately one child in every 2000 was autistic. Today the Center for Disease Control tells us the number has leaped to 1 in every 150. Could the use of heavy metals in vaccines be the culprit or has awareness increased with the advent of drugs like Ritalin?

Dr. Chris Exley, Ph.D. has dedicated two decades of his life into research on aluminum toxicity. Aluminum is the most common mineral on the planet. Dr. Exley believes it has been the mining and its subsequent usage that has led to the rise in neurological disorders. He has also found a simple solution and that is another mineral, silica. Silica has been refined out of most food products. We don't get enough of it in the diet. You might find it in a Health Food Store but it comes under the cosmetic end of things as ladies use it to improve complexion. Exley had a small test group of children who improved significantly when given silica and a further study of 15 adults suffering from Alzheimer's disease were given a liter of "*Spritzer Water*" (a Malaysian brand high in silica) for 13 weeks. Aluminum levels were lower by between 50-70% in all the test subjects. Deterioration in 8 of the 15 ceased altogether and 3 showed significant cognitive improvement. Mineral waters high in ionic silicic acid will reduce aluminum toxicity because they can penetrate the blood brain barrier. Both Fiji and Volvic Water have high ionic silica levels.

Treatment using Volvic/Fiji Water to Lower Blood/Brain Aluminum Levels:

Drink one 1.5 liter bottle of either Fiji or Volvic water daily for 5 days. Drink the entire bottle within an hour. Continue drinking Volvic/Fiji water on a regular basis. The aluminum will be excreted through the urine. Along with the water take 1 tablespoon of Extra Virgin Coconut Oil daily. Let's go ahead and kill two birds with one stone:

"Dr. Mary Newport runs a neo-natal ward in a Florida hospital but her interest in the coconut began not in her work environment but in her home. Her husband, Steve, was diagnosed with Alzheimer's disease after a poor showing on the traditional clock test used to signal the disease. Patients are asked to draw a clock showing a numbered face and hands

capable of demonstrating time. Steve performed so poorly that he was described as having severe symptoms. He had been withdrawing both socially and emotionally during the two years prior to diagnosis. It had also been difficult for him to read and he found he could no longer run. Mary was scared when she witnessed what was happening to her husband. So she set about studying Alzheimer's and was determined to find a way to help improve her husband's failing health. She explored the disease and found that it was best described as a diabetes of the brain. The culprit she discovered is the hormone insulin, manufactured by the beta islet cells of the pancreas. In the case of Alzheimer's, because of the insulin problem, the brain cells stop accepting glucose. Glucose is the principal brain food, and when cells begin to starve they start to die. When this occurs, there is an alternative food that remains acceptable, and this is ketones. Insulin, a storage hormone, sweeps glucose into the liver where it changes to glycogen and is stored as an energy source. This means when the sugar supply expires, the liver changes fats to ketones. This is one reason that people who fast on a "Detox Program" lose weight. They stop eating, so glucose dries up and then the body has to start burning its own fat deposits as an alternative fuel.

Dr. Newport found that long chain fatty acids like Coconut Oil provided the necessary fats for the ketone process to happen. She then started adding pure, non-hydrogenated Coconut Oil to her husband's diet and was astonished to see an improvement in just two short weeks. It was then he re-did the clock test and the result was noticeably better. He also became more talkative and less emotionally detached. After a month, he was able to run again, and the ability to read came back to him, too. She was so delighted with the results that she decided to write: "Alzheimer's Disease; What If There Was a Cure?", and share this new knowledge with other people. She received an encouraging response with feedback messages flooding in from family members awestruck with the improvements they were seeing in their loved ones.

Another issue raised its head. When the campaign to

denigrate fats as harmful to heart health emerged, the cholesterol myth began to appear. Anything that raised cholesterol was dammed and outed as dangerous. I have experienced such a response whilst talking to a physician from Europe. There are two types of cholesterol that are named after their transportation systems. One is LDL or Low-Density Lipoprotein, and the other is HDL that translates to High-Density Lipoprotein. LDL is said to be harmful and HDL is described as being healthful. Coconut Oil aligns itself with HDL, thus is by definition a healthy fat.

According to Dr. Beverly Teter of the University of Maryland, Coconut Oil improves the overall cholesterol factor in the body. She also found that it helped diminish the symptoms of Parkinson's disease, as well as Schizophrenia and acted as an antibiotic which can kill viruses. Conventional antibiotics don't destroy viruses although frequently they are mis-prescribed to do just that. Dr. Teter tells us that Coconut Oil helps boost the immune system, and it is this, meaning the body's defense system that is responsible for killing harmful pathogens."
Alister Bredee

What's the solution? We have already had one, actually two. You have recently completed a Kidney Cleanse. It was the first step in the program. You made a Parsley/Coriander tea that you drank every morning. Both herbs are powerful chelating agents. When a toxic metal like mercury or aluminum binds with a chelating agent, it's extracted from tissue and organs and excreted via the kidneys in the form of urine and through the intestinal tract in the form of stool. This initial cleanse *"served as a powerful heavy metal chelator"*. That is why I recommend repeating the *"Kidney Cleanse"* on a regular basis.

For the second step we look to the US Navy who in 1948 successfully used *"Ethylene-diamine-tetra-acetic acid"* (EDTA) as a chelator to overcome lead poisoning. EDTA chelation has grown to become very popular. It has dramatically improved conditions like arteriosclerosis; it has also improved symptoms associated with angina, gangrene and neuropathy, and has been instrumental in enhancing memory, improving vision as well as other sensory functions.

More about Silica

Silica improves collagen elasticity. That's why you will find it in the skin section of a *"Health Food Store"*. It ensures flexibility in all the body's connective tissues including the tendons and the cartilage. This reduces aches and pains and keeps you supple and your skin young and moist. But here's another thing. High levels of blood serum silica stop arterial plaque from clogging blood vessels. There has been a lot of huffing and puffing about how LDL cholesterol has been a major agent in the causation of sclerosis, but a more recent take has been focused on how serum calcium is the main culprit for arterial calcification. Without sufficient Sillca, Magnesium, Vitamin D3 and K2 as well as Calcium break off from the bones, especially in an acidic environment and remain in the blood and then can calcify in the soft tissue of the inner arteries and in the heart itself. Be sure then to take sufficient silica in your diet. Remember, it's a missing ingredient in most foods. Drinking water high in *"ionic silicic acid"*; we have already mentioned Volvic and Fiji Water, is imperative. There are others so check labels. In the UK Boots, the Chemist have a proprietary brand called *"Brecon Carreg"*; it contains 7% silica and boasts a pH of 7.6. Other non-water sources include the herb *'horsetail"*, *"cucumbers"* and *"diatomaceous earth powder"* (Fulvic Acid). The latter lack the ionic suspension of silicic acid found in the waters, as this can penetrate the blood/brain barrier. That means the water is better.

Toxic metals have been associated with new and emerging chronic illnesses, some of these we have already seen. Sadly we live on a poisoned planet. Environmental disregard has never been at such a high level. Industry has spewed over 6000 active synthetic compounds into the atmosphere, whilst industrial farming methods have added to the ever increasing problem.

In the USA in 1999, the Environmental Protection Agency found 20 out of the 29 fertilizers available in 12 States contained deadly metals that exceeded the designated limits. In 2001 the *"Environmental News Service"* reported that food grown with fertilizers containing more than the legal limit of heavy metals was ..."*the single greatest source of pollution exposure."*

Heavy Metal Detox

Certainly, EDTA, DMPS and DMSA mobilize and eliminate heavy metals quickly, but too quickly is not good; it stresses the body's *"detox"* pathways. The *"Cat Has Nine Lives And So Do You", h*eavy metal detox is a much gentler approach. You have already seen that simply drinking mineral water containing ionic silicic acid is an easy and powerful first step.

Activated Liquid Zeolite. The liquid form is more effective than the powdered variety. Zeolites are minerals that have a specific crystalline superstructure. They occur naturally in volcanic rock formations. Their honeycomb shaped cavities trap metals and toxins at a cellular level. The mineral is negatively charged, but most metals are positively charged. The negative charge pulls the positively charged metals to it, like a magnet. These particles are then trapped in the honeycomb structure. As the zeolite molecules grow heavier, the body cannot support the ensuing negative-positive energy charge occurring in the zeolite crevices. Such an interaction causes *"chaos"* which has no place in the system. Then the metal heavy zeolite molecule is expelled naturally via the urine. Zeolite is relatively slow acting, but reports from users are very positive. Conclusive results have been verified by hair analysis. If you feel that heavy metals are a particular problem, this is a recommended solution. Be patient as the metals are first released from fat tissue, then from the muscles and lastly from the bones. The latter hold onto heavy metals like uranium.

Start with 1 Drop in a glass of water. Go easily because at the outset you are likely to experience a detox reaction.

Week 2: 2 drops in water
Week 3: 3 drops in water
Week 4: 5 drops in water
Week 6: 7 drops in water
Week 8: 9 drops in water
Week 9: 10 drops in water
Week 11: 12 drops in water
Week 13: 15 drops in water
Week 14: 15 drops in water X2 a day
Week 15: 15 drops in water X3 a day. Maintain this dose until week 26.

**Warning: Minerals like magnesium, calcium, zinc and copper are all metals. They will be removed during the *"detox"*. To compensate for this be sure to take a good quality chelated multi- mineral supplement over the 26 weeks.

The site "Wellbeing Market Place"

http://www.wellbeingmarketplace.com/contents/en-us/d51.html

Offers many detox products. This is an Australian Company. They stock an acceptable form of liquid zeolite; it is enriched with Vitamins A and E to help with the process.

They also sell *"Detoxadine"* (nascent iodine). This helps support the thyroid, whilst promoting the removal of the halogens fluoride, chlorine and bromine. If you live in an area in which the water is fluoridated this might be useful for you. Most tap water is chlorinated by law in order to kill bacteria but bromine is another story. All these are powerful oxidizing agents, so they cause inflammation via free radical damage. Bromine used to be added to high octane petrol to stop the lead clogging the car's engine. Fortunately, that practice has stopped and it is now used principally as a fire retardant. There was a story that bromide used to be added to the tea in boarding schools to curb sexual urges. I don't know if that is true! However, I mention this in passing and make no recommendations. If you have a thyroid problem and a lot of people do.; this may be useful for you. If in doubt have the thyroid checked out.

Dentistry and Heavy Metals

Are there any amalgam fillings in your mouth? Mercury used in dentistry is extremely toxic. *"Silver fillings"*, as they are called (gets around the mercury issue), contain around 50% mercury. Dr. Joe Mercola tells us that a single dental amalgam filling releases as much as 15ug of mercury on a daily basis. Note this; scientists have issued a worldwide warning about mercury-containing seafood, with levels of between 2 and 3ug and yet people walk around with fillings emitting 5 times that amount and that's considered to be safe. There is something not right here, somewhere!

Charles Brown is President of *"The World Alliance of Mercury Free Dentistry"*. He says this:

"Amalgam is a primitive, polluting 19th Century product that began when physicians were sawing off legs! Medicine has since moved forward." The American Dental Association continues to use mercury and disputes the safety aspect. The height of irony is *"dental amalgam"* is shipped as a hazardous product to the dentist's premises and the leftover is also treated as hazardous.

There is no such thing as a safe mercury filling. I recommend, if you have them, you must have them removed, but they have to be taken out by a dentist who has been trained in a safe removal protocol. Using improper extraction techniques create huge health risks. Lots of mercury vapor is released during the process, this means special ventilation is necessary. As is a lot of other specialized equipment which *"untrained"* dentists don't usually have. I have personal experience of the dangers. I went to a dentist in Ireland who had been trained in *"mercury extraction"* in Australia. I had several mercury fillings which he agreed to remove and replace over a period of two months. We negotiated a set price for the work and then began; bear in mind you cannot deal with more than two teeth in any one session. However, he had a lot of difficulty with one tooth, which took over an hour to repair. This effected the agreed pricing structure. He was now behind in the work, so at the end, he rushed the process. He finished and I went on my merry way. Ten days later I became very ill. I developed a high fever and my glands swelled like balloons. I stayed in bed for a week and took large doses of Echinacea which fortunately reduced the swelling and the fever. Beware.....and make certain you select a *"Biological Dentist"* who has been specially trained in mercury removal. *"The International Academy of Biological Dentistry and Medicine"*, have a practitioner listing, which principally covers North America. In the UK *"The British Society for Mercury Free Dentistry"* also has a register whilst in Thailand, the *"Thantakit International Dental Centre"* offers treatment following safe removal guidelines. Some dentists will tell you they can remove amalgams, but be quite sure they have undergone specialized training before allowing any treatment to commence.

Every Tooth Connects to a Bodily Organ

We mentioned this earlier. Every one of the teeth in your head relates to a Chinese Medicine meridian as well as to a specific bodily organ.

For example tooth number 32 on the right-hand side of the lower jaw relates to the Heart and Small intestine meridians. A cavity here could well lead to right-sided shoulder pain. It could also lead to heart issues. If you have dental problems you need to take action. Don't delay, act right away! Find a good dentist, preferably someone who adopts a *"Holistic"* or *"Biological"* approach. Caries exist because teeth break down due to the presence of bacteria in the mouth. *"Streptococcus Mutans"* is the worst offender. An over acidic mouth environment causes bacteria to flourish. You see that nutrition plays a significant factor in dental health. Reducing your sugar intake is critical. Sugar acidifies the oral cavity causing the pH to decrease. As this happens the electrical voltage in the tooth drops. To increase pH the alkaline level needs to increase. Bicarbonate of soda is very alkaline. Using this as a cleaning agent is excellent, especially last thing at night before bed as it increases oral alkalinity and gives the teeth a fighting chance to resist decay. Oh, and don't forget to *"Oil Pull"* first thing in the morning!

Acumeridian Tooth-Organ Relationships

Acumeridian Tooth-Organ Relationships — from various sources including Gleditsch and Klinghardt (www.NeuralTherapy.com). Compiled by Dr. Ralph Wilson.

Figure 11

Decayed teeth lead to fillings, root canals and extractions. We have talked about fillings already. Be sure to have your amalgams removed and replaced with *"Composite resin which is the most common alternative to dental amalgam. Fillings like this are sometimes called "tooth-colored" or "white". Composite resin alternatives are made of a type of plastic (an acrylic resin) reinforced with powdered glass filler.*

Advantages of composite resin fillings include:

Blend in with surrounding teeth

High strength

Require minimal removal of healthy tooth structure for placement "(US Gov.)

Be very careful of root canals. A root canal entails the removal of the material in the middle and down to the root of the tooth. The purpose is to eradicate an immediate infection, but the end-result is often the opposite. Dr. Weston A. Price (1870-1948) was a leading authority on dental health. He determined many types of degenerative diseases were caused by root canals. These diseases include several forms of heart disorders, kidney and bladder maladies, arthritis, rheumatism, psychological illness, lung disease and differing forms of cancer. He was the Chairman and leading authority of the *"American Dental Association"* from 1914-1923. He published a two-volume study on the dangers of root canals and cavitations; work which was later taken up by Dr. Hal Huggins himself a controversial figure and fervent opponent of amalgam fillings.

If you have root canals you will find *"A Cat Has Nine Lives And So Do You",* is essential for your health and well-being. Root canals compromise the immune system. Immunity is challenged because you have dead tissue in your mouth. You need to boost the system to overcome the challenge. There are alternatives to root canals; implants are a case in question. However, the substitutes pose their own problems. For answers, it is best to talk to a "Biological Dentist". They oppose the presence of dead tissue in the mouth and will give you better options in order to find solutions that relate to your particular case.

Ultimately the answers to better oral and general health can be found in childhood. Once we are here we might take a quick look at toothpaste. The recent Cornucopia report "Behind the Dazzling Smile" outlines risk behind several toothpaste ingredients. Fluoride, of course, raises its ugly head. Make no mistake it's a poison, but it has long been heralded as the answer to decaying teeth. A 2010 study found the supposedly helpful fluorapatite layers to be 6 nanometers thick. This is infinitesimal; so thin it is quickly destroyed by chewing. The Saji Company of Japan has come up with a miraculous sounding product that they claim will soon make dentists redundant. It's Apagard Nano hydroxyapatite remineralizing toothpaste. This fluoride free product claims to re-build teeth. Feedback has been very positive, so much so that the American Dental Association has lobbied to have it removed from the American market!

Other research has shown the cacao extract 'theobromine" repairs and re-mineralizes dentin far more effectively. Better to buy 85% or more cacao chocolate than fancy toothpastes full of health damaging chemicals. Natural toothpastes are available. Check them out. You can if you choose make your own.

Natural Toothpaste Recipe

Take two tablespoons of coconut oil, add enough sodium bicarbonate to give the oil a solid consistency. You may add a couple of drops of peppermint essential oil to give the mixture a pleasant smell. Store in a glass container. Clean teeth night and morning and after meals.

Good diet, as pointed out by Dr. Weston Price plays a pivotal role.

Be sure to have a generous intake of Vitamin C, D3 and K2 (comes from green leafy vegetables and fermented foods).

Magnesium (at least 500 mg daily)

Phosphorous (found in pumpkin seeds, Brazil nuts, fish and

certain meats)

Potassium and Calcium. (Potassium is found in fruit and vegetables.

Diets made acidic by high sugar and carbohydrate content destroy teeth. Maybe it's too late for you, but ensure your children eat well and their teeth should last them for the rest of their lives.

An Alkalizing Remedy

Take a fresh lemon, preferably organic.

A liter of spring water

A package of Sodium Bicarbonate. This is not Baking Soda which is a different product often containing aluminum. Purchase from the pharmacy, not the supermarket.

Squeeze the lemon into the water and add 1 tablespoon of Sodium Bicarbonate ($NaHCO_3$). Place the mixture in the fridge overnight.

Drink one glass first thing in the morning and another before bed at night. If you are highly acidic due to diet and excessive coffee and alcohol consumption you might experience stomach cramps and loose at the outset. Don't worry they will pass. Then you can increase your intake to 2 and then 3 glasses first thing every morning. Continue the therapy for a month, take the next month off and so on.

Life 7 – The Emotional Detox

I don't care if you claim to have had the most idyllic of childhoods but I am willing to bet the bank on the fact you still have trapped emotions lurking somewhere in the subconscious mind. Those emotions need to be released in order for you to completely detoxify. The trapped emotions steal energy and take the joy out of living. People who claim this is *"not so"* are in denial. They need this work more than anybody else.

The Amazing Subconscious Mind

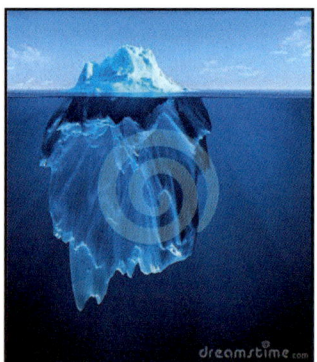

Figure 12

The mind is best described when it's compared to an iceberg. 10% of the *"ice mountain"* lies above the surface and 90% lies hidden beneath. The visible 10% matches the *"conscious mind"*. We fool ourselves when we think this one is in charge." It can cope with the maximum of 10 actions at any one time. Some are not so adept and find it difficult to whistle and walk down the street at the same time. The *"subconscious mind"* is a very different story. It can process up to 15,000,000 bits of information per second. That is far superior to any computer yet invented. It runs your body, it stores your memories, and it's the home of your emotions. It can make you sick and it can make you well. It's utterly fantastic! Its highest prime directive is to keep you safe. If you ae alive and well whilst reading this, then it has done a good job. Doesn't it deserve a big thank-you?

Communicating with the subconscious can be problematic, however. There are ways. Meditation is one and hypnosis another. This is where we lift the conscious mind, sitting on top of all the multitudinous aspects that lie underneath. Dreams are a valuable indicator of what is going on in the subconscious. Freud wrote a book called *"The Royal Road to the Unconscious"*, explaining this. However, it was the chiropractors who met in Chicago in the 1960s who came up with another means. Because *"muscle testing"* is a very efficient tool for discovering material buried in the subconscious.

As we have just said there are many ways to establish the presence of these lurking emotions; muscle testing is particularly useful. A muscle test is a bio-feedback device, which gives information from the bio-computer (subconscious mind). Another way of describing this would be to call it the body-mind mix. Muscle testing is the language of Kinesiology, which was developed by George Goodheart and other chiropractors in the 1960s. The reason Kinesiology emerged was because the chiropractors were having problems getting their adjustments to hold. Far too often a chiropractor worked on a patient, only to find the adjustment he had made came "unglued" very shortly afterwards. Goodheart developed *"Applied Kinesiology"* to address this problem and get information from the body to help find the answers. The subconscious is simply amazing. It knows the difference between *"yes'* and *"no"*. It works a bit like a "polygraph" or lie detector test. The polygraph shows a subtle, yet measurable bodily response when questioned. A muscle test demonstrates a similar but more amplified reaction. Strength shows *"truth"* or *"yes"* or a positivity. A weak response would be *"no"* or a negativity.

Muscle testing done gently is about the subtle changes taking place in your own body (self-testing) or in somebody else's. It serves as the beginner's guide to intuition. Think of it as inner awareness with training wheels. Some say that intuition is the voice of God. Listen carefully and be guided by this still, small voice within.

The Sway Test

The easiest way to get the feel of muscle testing, which is simply a means of establishing communication with the subconscious is to spend some time practicing the *"sway test"*. It's really very easy. It's an *"ideomotor test"*; meaning an idea or thought connects with a motor response, even if the idea or thought lies at the subconscious level. To do the *"sway test"*, you use the whole standing body. Just as a tree leans to face the sun, the human body inclines, naturally towards aspects that agree with it. If something is beneficial the body will incline in that direction, if it is harmful it will recoil in the opposite direction. This is a great test to use when you are out shopping in the supermarket and would like some guidance in knowing which of the tomatoes on display are the best buy. Here's how it works:

Think *"yes"* with a strong positive feeling. Pause, step out of the head and let the body move freely of its own accord. A positive *"yes"* will cause your body to sway slightly forward. Try it ......and see. Repeat a few times for practice.

Think *"no"*, with a *"yucky"* negative feeling. Notice the response. It will lean slightly backwards or to the side. Try it a few times. That is a demonstration of an "ideomotor" response.

Let's go through it again. This time in more detail. To begin find your point of balance.

You do this by placing the feet firmly on the ground and sway backwards and forwards until you find your center of gravity. It's a *"teeter-totter"* point of equilibrium.

Now say the word *"yes"*. What happens? Does your body fall backwards or forwards?

It should move forwards. If you fall backwards you might be

reversed. Tap your thymus for the duration of a breath and try again. Reversal means *"chi"* or Meridian energy is flowing backwards.

Now say the word *"no"*. Do you move backwards or forwards? You should move backwards, or perhaps sideways. If not tap the thymus and try again.

Congratulations... you have established a *"yes"*, *"no"* level of communication with the subconscious.

It's time now move to slightly more complex issues. Start with this sentence. *"My name is_____* (add your name). Does your body move backwards or forwards? It should move forwards.

Now say "M*y name is_____* (give another name). What happens now? Do you move backwards or forwards?

Try experimenting with several true/ false statements. A little practice will soon get you using the technique easily.

OK you are ready for the $1,000, 000 question. *"I have some trapped emotions?"* *"Yes"* or *"No"*.

If the answer is *"yes"*. Ask *"How many?"* *"One"*, *"two"*, *"three"*, *"four"* etc. Proceed until you get a *"no"* *The number before the "no" is the total.* This is what we have to work with. Write down the number.

Emotional issues are the basis of most health concerns. According to Dr. Geerd Hamer, the founder of *"Germanic New Medicine"*, who states categorically that all illness starts with a causative event which creates the trapped emotion. Dr. Hamer is an oncologist. His son. Dirk, was shot dead in the late 1970's. Two years later Dr. Hamer developed testicular cancer and felt there had to be a connection. Fortunately there was a ward full of cancer patients to work with, and they confirmed his findings. In all cases, there was a causative incident 1-4 years before diagnosis. This he called the DHS (Dirk Hamer Syndrome...after his son). The reaction created a lesion on the brain. The lesion can be detected by CT scan. The doctor has more than 30,000 CT scans to prove his point. Remove the causative trapped emotion(s) and then a true healing can be facilitated.

What are Trapped Emotions?

During moments of intense emotion the energy of the emotion becomes trapped. It will always lodge somewhere, usually in the trunk of the body. But it can stick anywhere.

Trapped emotions can occur at any age or can even be inherited.

They cause inflammation, pain, congestion, self-sabotage, depression, phobias etc.

They are things and have the size of an orange or bigger.

They distort the normal energy field

All trapped emotions are lodged within the Chinese Meridian System.

By releasing these emotions we set in motion a powerful healing process. The initial work needs to be completed with a competent therapist, who has the skill and objectivity to see to the heart of the issue. Please talk to us here at:

Healthambitconsultancy@protonmail.com

To set up a session and to make recommendations for this work to be done effectively for you.

After you have cleared the *"bigger* issues it is very important that you learn a simple technique that you can use yourself to address the day-to-day concerns that pop up in life. That means you can take care of yourself, and only need to recourse to a therapist in times of extreme crisis. These should be few and far between when you are equipped with some simple tools you can use yourself!

The tapping techniques that fall under the heading of *"Meridian Energy Techniques"*, are straightforward, easy to administer and above all effective.

The State of Energy Psychology Research

"Energy psychology (EP) modalities have been researched by more than 100 investigators in at least 7 countries. As of 2016, over 60 research studies have been published on EP modalities; out of these only one has not shown efficacy.

The results of these studies have been published in more than 15 different peer-reviewed journals, including the *Journal of Clinical Psychology,* the *Journal of Nervous and Mental Disease* and the APA journals *Psychotherapy: Theory, Research, Practice, Training* and *Review of General Psychology.* While many important questions remain to be answered, a great deal of groundwork is in place.

The next frontier of EP research involves exploring the mechanisms of action of these modalities and investigating concurrent physiological changes using such tools as DNA microarrays (gene chips), MEGs (magnetoencephalograms), fMRI and PET scans and neurotransmitter and hormone assays."

All the Meridian Techniques evolved from the work of American Clinical Psychologist Dr. Roger Callahan. Dr. Callahan went to study *"Kinesiology"* in the 1970s. Psychologists simply did not study *"body-work"* procedures at that time; this was a radical departure. He knew about the *"Meridian System"* and how *"chi"* circulated in the body. This made him admirably prepared for his *"client"* Mary. She had been visiting him at his home-office in Palm Springs for the best part of two years, because of her extreme fear of water. The work they had done together over time meant she had progressed from a fear state where it was hard for her to go out in the rain or have a bath, to one of discomfort, where she was able to move out and sit on the deck beside his swimming pool. On the fateful day in question, she arrived for her session complaining about a stomach ache. Callahan knew from his studies that the acupoint just below the eye is *"stomach 1".* Namely, the beginning point on the stomach meridian which extends down to the second toe. He tapped her on this point for a few seconds, hoping to ease her pain. She leaped up and began to move quickly towards the pool, yelling as she went, *it's gone!"* Her psychologist was alarmed, knowing she could not swim. *"It's*

OK!" she laughed. *"The fear, it's gone!"* Dr. Callahan had stumbled on something, and that was how "Meridian Energy Psychology" was born.

The foundation statement of what was to become T.F.T. (Thought Field Therapy) and later morph into E.F.T. (Emotional Freedom Technique) states:

"All negative emotions and limiting beliefs create a disruption in the body's energy field."

TFT was popular with members of the *"psycho-therapeutic"* profession because the simple process of tapping on the end points of acupuncture meridians was quick and easy and produced effective results. One of the therapists who attended Dr. Callahan's training was Clinical Psychologist Dr. Larry Nims. He developed one of the simplest and most user-friendly variants of the *"tapping techniques"*. It's called "BE SET FREE FAST", BSFF for short. The name is an acronym:

BE SET = Behavioral and Emotional Symptom Elimination Training

FAST = Fear, Anger, Sadness and Trauma. I have added a 5th emotion, which is Limitation.

The technique delves to the emotional roots of a problem. These comprise a collection of gestalts (strings) which are impressed into the subconscious. The subject taps on 5 acupuncture meridian end points whilst focusing on the issue being treated. When meridians are tapped in this way, a small electrical charge is sent down the channel. Placing a needle in an acupoint does a similar thing. The small charge restores the energetic balance. It's a bit like repairing a blown fuse. None of this is an intellectual exercise. We are not analyzing the problem, but accessing the feelings generated by the issue. *"The Course of Miracles,"* tells us that there are only two emotions, love at one end of the spectrum and fear at the other. Everything else is a variant of the two basics. Frankly, I believe that simplification to be too complex. I believe there are only two feelings. They are light and heavy. If something feels heavy, cramped, dull, constricted, restricted unpleasant, it's somewhere we don't want to be. On the other hand, if we have a place that is bright, light, breezy, expansive, and comfortable, a position in which we feel at home, which would you rather have? It's a no-brainer, isn't it? After treatment people usually say the matter has become lighter (better), the same (more work needed) or remains heavy (no change). Let's be realistic, don't expect to turn a negative feeling full circle or 180* in one simple tapping round. If the feelings become lighter persist until all heaviness has disappeared entirely. You might have to repeat the process several times, but the ensuing light, bright, expansive result is well worth the effort. Again BSFF is a simple technique, but utterly useless if you don't use it whenever it's required.

Daily Clearing Session

I suggest everybody schedules 10 minutes daily for a clearing session. Take time to reflect on issues. If anything is *"bothersome"*, clear it. Done repeatedly this will change your life.

These are the steps:

First take a look at the diagram to locate the tapping points.

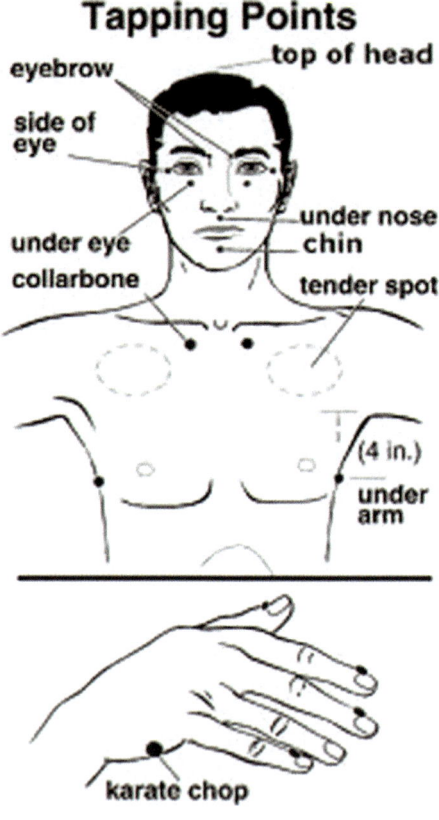

Figure 13

The points you are going to use are:
- The eyebrow point (end of eyebrow)
- Under eye point (bone directly under the eye)
- The inside edge of the little finger (See hand

diagram)

- The inside edge of the ring finger. That's the finger next to the "pinkie".
- The Outside edge of the first finger.

Tap the points with one or two fingers. All acupoints are bilateral. (We exclude central and governing strange flows because they are not really meridians. Moreover, they are not relevant here!)

You can tap on the left, on the right or on both sides. Tap the points whilst thinking of the issue causing discomfort and repeating the wording as laid out.

BSFF Formula (adapted)

Tap on eyebrow point: (Bladder 2) and say:
"I am eliminating all of the sadnesses in all of the roots and the deepest cause of all of this problem."

Tap under the eye (stomach 1) and say:
"I am eliminating all of the fears in all of the roots and the deepest cause of all of this problem."

Tap on the inside edge of the little finger (Heart 9) and say:
"I am eliminating all of the angers in all of the roots and the deepest cause of all of this problem."

Tap on the inside edge of the ring finger (Triple Warmer 1) and say:
"I am eliminating all of the limitations in all of the roots and the deepest cause of all of this problem."

Tap on the eyebrow points (Bladder 2) and say:
"I am eliminating all of the emotional traumas in all of the roots and the deepest cause of all of this problem."

If appropriate treat for forgiveness:
Tap on outside edge of the first finger (Large Intestine 1) and

say:

"I forgive you (Mum, Dad, John, or whoever) and I know that you are/were doing the best you could with the resources you have/had.

For God say: "I forgive you God (or whatever term you use) and I know that you are/were always there and doing the best and right thing for me."

For the world or for life say: "I forgive you world/life and I know that you are just being what you are."

"I forgive myself and I know I am/was doing the best I can/could."

Forgiveness

....or The Terrible Cost of Unforgiveness

By Psychologist Larry Phillip Nims, Ph.D., creator of BSFF-Be Set Free Fast

http://www.besetfreefast.com

"Historically, forgiveness has been addressed rather minimally and ineffectively in traditional therapies. We have always recognized that unforgiveness was a problem in human adjustment. But, we have tended largely to ignore it as a treatment issue.

There are many reasons for such neglect I suppose, not the least of which is that we really were not sure how to eliminate it. Another is that many of us are uncomfortable and/or unfamiliar with spiritual considerations in psychotherapy.

Roger Callahan pointed the way for the technical process of treating unforgiveness. He deserves much credit for this finding. Still, he did not seem to recognize and/or acknowledge the enormity of the negative effects of unforgiveness on the human soul and spirit.

Here are just some of the inevitable costs to you and me whenever we hold onto unforgiveness. They are all in operation, continuously, in every unforgiveness, whether we consciously recognize them or not. These consequences happen within everyone every time that we get entrapped in unresolved unforgiveness. We have all paid these high costs in our lives over and over again. We probably still do pay them in many unhealed areas of our psyches and our spirits.

Consider these consequences of judgment, criticism and unforgiveness.

We continue to feel the psychological pain of the perceived offense.

We block healthy communication and potential reconciliation with the "offender".

We perceive similar offenses by others who remind us of the offender.

We attract similar situations, people and injuries to ourselves.

We give up our personal power to others to determine how we will feel and respond (actually, we "react") in similar situations.

We render ourselves incapable of ever really knowing, and learning from, the full truth about the event that damaged the relationship.

We take added toxic negativity into our present relationships.

We isolate/prevent/avoid/limit ourselves from having new, more healthy, and more fulfilling relationships.

We become vulnerable to becoming spiteful, resentful and bitter.

We disrespect, distrust and devalue ourselves at deep levels of our psyches.

We block ourselves spiritually from receiving help and healing from our Higher Source.

Our own spirits and souls "shrivel up" (contract) more and more.

Yet, most of us have some of these attitudes buried deep within our subconscious minds. I have not seen a client yet who does not have numerous unresolved hurts and other emotional injuries, always with judgment, criticism, unforgiveness and related negative attitudes attached.

Fortunately, we now have the tools and the therapeutic support no longer to be victimized in all of these ways by the devastation of anger and unforgiveness. We can readily neutralize and eliminate all of the psychological, but not the spiritual, costs of unforgiveness simply by treating ourselves with BSFF.

Here is how:

Resolving Anger and Unforgiveness with BSFF-Be Set Free Fast Whenever you finish a session of any energy therapy treatment, remember to treat for anger and unforgiveness toward yourself or anyone else, including God if that is an issue, for every problem you have just treated. Do this after every session of BSFF treatments, whether you have just done one or a 101 treatments in that session.

You can do just one treatment for all angers combined for each person you were angry at, one treatment for all angers toward God, and one treatment for all angers toward yourself. You do not have to treat anger for each incident, although you may choose to in some instances. Just make sure that you treat separately for every person that you were angry at in the session of BSFF treatments you have just completed.

Always be sure to treat angers before going to unforgiveness. Remember that anger gives rise to judgment, criticism and related hurtful attitudes and these give rise to unforgiveness. So treat them in that order.

The most important reason for doing this work at the end of a session of treatments is to set ourselves free of the terrible effects of judgment, criticism, and any other related attitudes such as vengeance, wanting to harm or cause pain to someone or to put ourselves in a one-up position with someone else.

Taking such a superior attitude with the intention of causing harm or loss to someone, including oneself, is a major spiritual problem as well as a psychological problem. Consider this. When I take a judgmental, critical, punitive, vengeful or withholding position toward someone, including myself, what am I doing *spiritually? Well, I am playing God!*

Whether you view this violation from another religious or philosophical perspective or not, it still boils down to making myself the power and the center of the universe. That is a very dangerous position to be in because none of us has that power or authority in ourselves. It is reserved to our Higher Power. So, this is a losing battle for us--with all of the terrible costs described above.

So, always treat the angers first. This will also eliminate the judgment, criticalness and related negative attitudes that lead to unforgiveness. Then do the unforgiveness step. Notice that, if you try to do unforgiveness without eliminating the anger first, these negative attitudes will draw you back into the unforgiveness, sometimes almost immediately. So you are still on precarious ground.

You must treat anger at each person separately, but you may simultaneously treat all anger toward any specific person for all perceived hurts, offenses or failures that you addressed in that session by using just one BSFF sequence at the end of the session. Likewise, you can combine in one treatment all the unforgiveness toward any one person for everything you have just treated about that person during that session.

Be sure to always treat anger at self-last. If you do not do so, you will have to treat yourself again for anger at yourself for the related problems of anger, judgment, criticism and unforgiveness that you treat after you forgave yourself the first time in the session. No percentage in that is there? In other words, treat yourself last, so you will have covered all of your anger at self for all of the problems that you have just treated.

The marvelous payoff for doing this forgiveness work is that you completely eradicate all of the terrible costs in less than 15 seconds! Forgive everyone and enjoy the blessings of the wonderful new freedom you will have!"

Thank you, Larry Nims. Isn't that worth it?

After all, that tapping, do you now feel lighter or heavier?

I hope it's a lot lighter.

After TFT came...

EFT (Emotional Freedom Technique)

This was the brainchild of Gary Craig. Here is a simplified variant of this technique. Personally, I find this very powerful. Try in on an issue and discover for yourself.

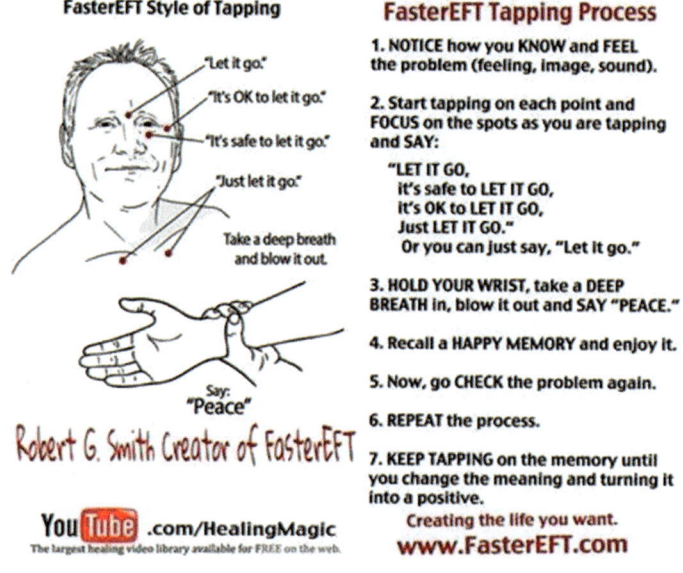

Figure 14

Life 8 – Energetic Toxicities

Yes, we are now talking about the energy waves that pass seen and unseen through our world. The immense explosion of cell phone usage over the last 20 years is staggering. I remember my first cell phone in the early 90's. It was the size of a brick. It was by no means the earliest variant of its type. Mobile phones are really radio transmitters and receivers, and this technology dates back before World War 11. Mine was a 2G model. The "G" stands for generation, and at that point, the industry took off. Today my *"brick"* phone is a dinosaur, but between 1984 and 2004 the second billion were spawned. In the following 18 months, the third billion shot onto the market. In 2016 2.082 billion people are said to be using "smartphones", regardless of the older devices that are still around. In third world countries, you will find the poorest of villagers the proud possessors of a cell phone.

In Sri Lanka, for example, a *"smartphone"* will cost the equivalent of what a junior teacher earns in a month. To pay for the luxury somebody would have to take out a high-interest bank loan, repayable over 3 years. Asides from the costs, this is a new technology, and nobody really knows the impact this will have on overall health, worldwide.

Dr. George Carlo, a health scientist, and epidemiologist headed a $28,000,000 program funded by the cell phone industry between 1993 -1998. When his research found adverse biological effects such as DNA damage and cancer, his funding was swiftly cut off. He claims that every study done has shown some evidence of health hazards. Many of these studies have been sponsored by the mobile phone industry itself and may not be entirely unbiased in their findings. With this gigantic explosion in usage ambient cell phone radiation has increased by 5000% in urban areas. How can we possibly gauge the effects of this particularly over time?

Are Mobile Phones Really Safe?

"On the 26th of June 1996, Irish investigative journalist, Veronica Guerin was fatally shot as her car paused at a red traffic light on Dublin's Naas Road. Guerin, one-time personal assistant to Irish Prime Minister Charlie Haughey had trained as an accountant before entering journalism, so she was well qualified to research the dealings of the drug gangs who had a fearsome reputation in Dublin's inner city. At her post-mortem, they found severe burns in the region of Guerin's right ear. As a journalist, she was a heavy user of the mobile phone. This posed some momentary questions about the safety of these devices.

The technology that made handheld mobiles possible was developed in the 1970s. Commercialization of the technology appeared in the 1980s and the expectation in the United Kingdom was skeptical with an anticipation of 10,000 phones selling worldwide. This figure was way off the mark. In 2006 international shipments exceeded one billion; it was estimated in 2010 that there were 5.2 billion cell phones in operation on the planet. The calculated world population is just over 7 billion. It would, therefore, be safe to postulate that market penetration has been enormously successful. In some countries, it exceeds 100%!

A mobile or cell phone is a small radio. They are called cell phones because for the radio to operate it has to broadcast its signal to cell towers. Most places have been divided up into cells of approximately 10 square miles in radius. The different phone companies all have a "Mobile Telephone Switching Office" in every population area. It is from here the signal is fed to the numerous transmission towers that dot the landscape. The system works because every phone company has a specific five figure identification number called a SID. When a device is turned on regardless of whether you are making a call or not it is constantly picking up the SID that is being beamed from the nearest tower. The mobile phone company is also transmitting to your phone a signal on specific channels that it is programmed to tune into. In Thailand, the situation is relatively lax (but no longer); in some countries, you have to register the phone with your personal details. That means the whereabouts of the user can be tracked.

With five billion sets worldwide; the mobile phone as an electrical device; emits photons creating an electromagnetic field. The electronic radiation is in the high-frequency microwave range. In effect, the caller is holding the equivalent of a microwave oven to the ear whilst chatting. No wonder Veronica Guerin had burn marks on the right side of her brain! Numerous studies have produced contradictory results. But many experts consider the risks related to phone usage to be very real indeed!

The World Health Organization has categorized mobile phones into group 2b on the IRAC scale. This gives them the dubious tag of being "possibly carcinogenic". The report continued by saying that further research was required.

We live in a wireless-saturated environment surrounded by modulated frequencies that are growing ever more complex due to the information that is being transmitted to mobile and smartphones as well as the all-pervasive Wi-Fi network. The ensuing EMFs are largely untested, and nobody really knows what the effect of all this electronic smog is having on the human population. Olle Johannsson of Stockholm's Karolinska Institute claims we are in the midst of "the largest full-scale experiment ever." The question that remains to be answered is what happens when we allow ourselves to be whole body irradiated by new EMFS, 24 hours per day for the rest of our lives?

Published media reviews are contradictory. Much of the research is carried out by the mobile phone industry and not surprisingly the results are skewed in their favor. Already we know that the risk of getting a brain tumor on the side of the head where the phone is placed increases by 40% for adults. Even more disturbing data calculates the rate of getting a cancer increase fivefold for those who started using mobiles before the age of 20.

In order to protect ourselves a little, it is better to limit cell phone use. Keep conversations brief and to the point. You can always use a landline for the longer and more personal calls. Or a better idea is to use a hands-free connection, which means you do not have to hold a microwave device next to the head. Have you ever asked yourself why your ear grows hot after a long chat?

As far as the ever growing waves that penetrate our bodies, you can protect yourself by buying Q-link pendants or Orgonite protectors that are available locally. Oh, be sure to switch the Wi-Fi off overnight!"

Alister Bredee

Here are Some More Considerations

- The weaker the reception the more power the phone uses. Avoid usage when the signal is weak.
- Avoid carrying the phone on your body, particularly in your breast or trouser pocket. Keep it in a bag and off your person.
- Do not sleep with a mobile phone under the pillow or near your head. Better still leave it outside the bedroom.
- Used a well-shielded wired headset.
- Limit your cell phone usage. Keep calls short. Send text messages where possible.
- Spend less time on apps. Use a laptop or notebook instead.

- Do not use the phone whilst eating. The low-level EMFs affect digestion.
- Frequent "smartphone' usage increases cortisol levels. It's a stressor.
- Don't let children use mobile phones. They are most susceptible to the dangers of low-level radiation.
- Switch off modems at night.
- Finally, buy some protection to stop the low-level EMF non-ionizing radiation. Orgonite makes an excellent protector. It's made from metal crystals and organic resin.

Orgonite is the brainchild of Wilhelm Reich.

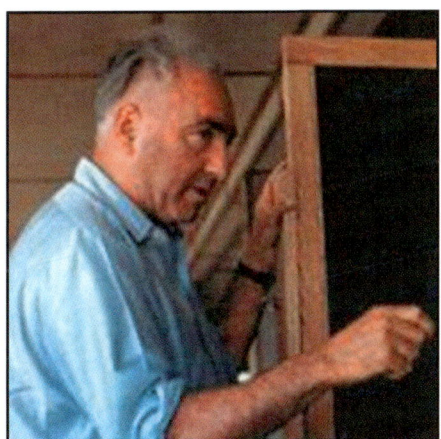

Figure 15

He was a contemporary of Freud and a noted psychotherapist in his own right; he is, however, better known for his research in bio-physics. In the 1930s he noticed an *"energetic connection that linked all living creatures. He called this "orgone energy"*. He worked until his death in 1957 demonstrating the laws and manifestation of this. He showed *"orgone radiation"* to be similar to the energy given off by the sun. Further experiments indicated this ever present energy would be repelled by metal objects and absorbed by organic material. By making a box with alternate layers of organic material (wood) and inorganic (metal), he found he would accumulate a more concentrated field of *"orgone"*. He called these boxes *"orgone accumulators"* and used them to great effect to treat cancer patients.

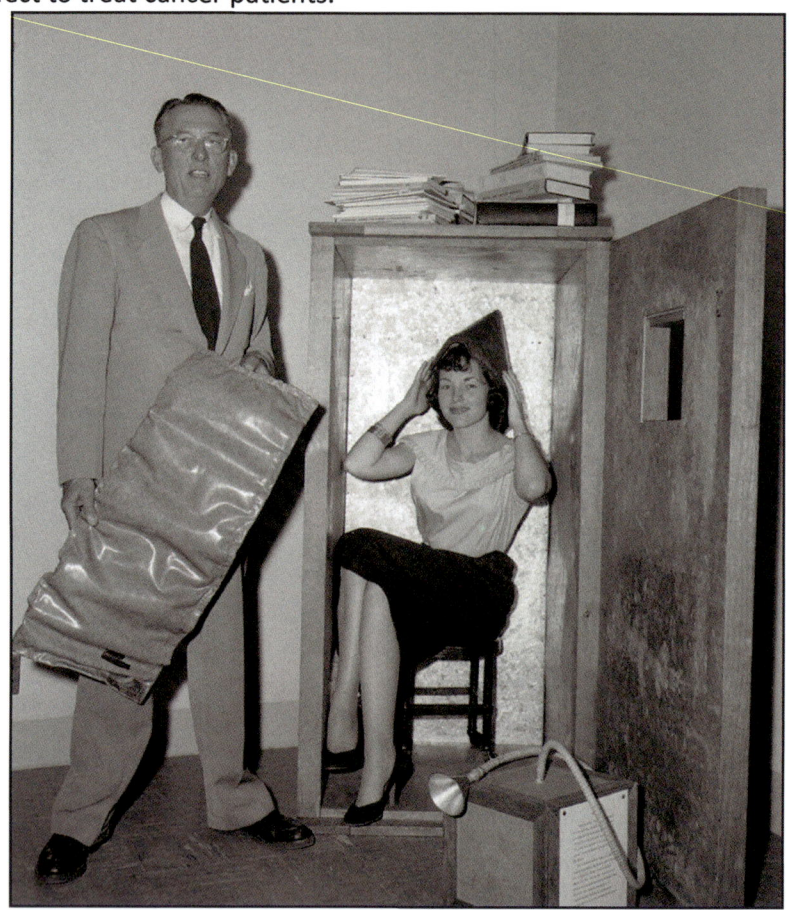

Figure 16

Today, "Orgonite" is made from metal in some form molded into an organic base, usually "fiberglass".

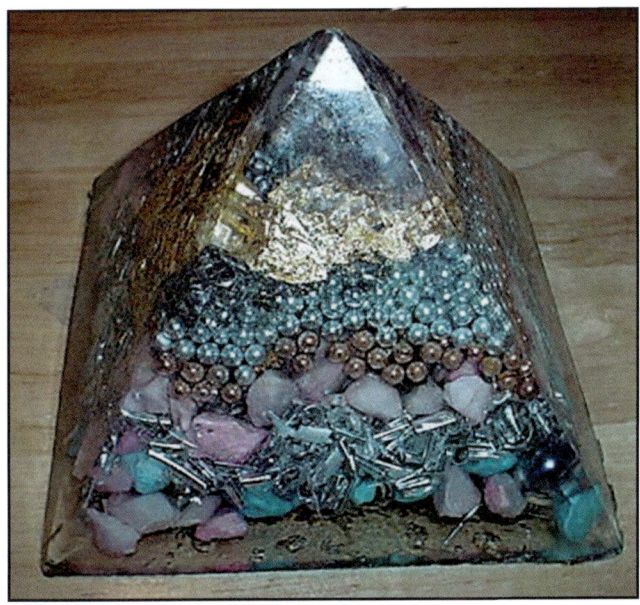

Figure 17

The resulting whole creates a "piezoelectric "effect. It seems the microwave energy coming off devices like mobile phones is chaotic in nature. This would be described by Reich as DOR (Deadly Organic Radiation). Orgonite does not reduce the radiation, but it stabilizes the DOR, turning it back into harmless *"orgone energy"*. The damage done by cell phones and similar devices is the result of the extremely low magnetic field generated on the electronic scale. It seems *"Orgonite"* works to reverse that damage. People who use the *"Orgonite"* devices usually report improved sleep and more energy. When exposed to harmful non-ionizing radiation, muscles test weak, but when protected by "Orgonite" they become strong once again.

Dr. Martin Black Ph.D., is a retired professor from Columbia University, in a talk, he gave entitled *"The Health Effects of Electromagnetic Fields"*, said, "the coiled structure of DNA is very vulnerable to EMFs!" It is not the heat that causes the harm, but the radiation itself. The National Toxicology Program (NTD) did a study on the effects of radio frequencies on rats which were exposed to cell phone radiation for 9 hours per day, 7 days per week for 2 years (the approximate lifespan of a rat). 2/3% of the males developed malignant gliomas and a further 5/7% developed nerve cell tumors of the heart. In humans, it seems it can take up to 10 years before symptoms show up.

If like me you are concerned about the news stories telling of the severe reduction in the honey-bee population, then what follows will be alarming. We have been told the reason for the disappearance has been blamed on pesticides, insecticides, disease and global warming. The true reason, however, rests with a mineral called *"magnetite"*. Early direction finding compasses comprised this lodestone. A piece of *"magnetite"* suspended on a string will show due north. The Chinese used this method to develop the earliest compasses as long ago as 300BC. Bees have *"magnetite"* in their intestines and birds in their beaks. This helps them find their way *"home"* by aligning them with the Earth's Magnetic Grid. This explains how *"homing pigeons"* can cover hundreds of miles to successfully find their way back to their hutch to safely deliver a message. This was an effective and efficient means of communication at the time of the Battle of Waterloo, 175 years before the mass advent of cell phones!

The market saturation of devices using low-level non-ionizing radiation to serve as a means of communication has put paid to homing pigeons…

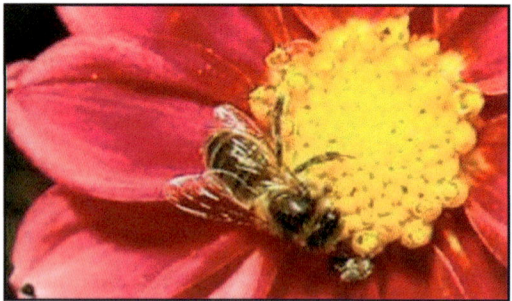

Figure 18

...and to honey bees, because it prevents the *"magnetite"* from aligning correctly with the magnetic grid of Mother Earth. The result; the birds and the bees get lost! This is disastrous; bees pollinate an immense amount of our food supply. According to the US Department of Agriculture, $1/3$ of the human diet is derived from pollinated plants, whilst the honey-bee is responsible for 80% of this pollination. That means we could all starve to death because of our fascination with the mobile phone. If *"they"* want to reduce the world's population here is one very effective way of achieving that objective! Eugenics to one side, I look at my *"smartphone"* with increased respect and use it only when truly necessary.

What about microwaves? We have read here about microwave radiation and many people use microwave ovens. I suspect it is impossible to avoid "microwaved" food especially if you eat out in public places. *Microwaves alter food for the worst!*

Hans Hertel conducted a serious study into the effects of microwaved food in the early 1990s. His small but well-controlled investigation showed conclusively that *"microwave cooking"* changes the nutrients in food and those changes were reflected in blood samples. He worked with Bernard H. Blanc of *"The Swiss Federal Institute of Technology"*. The results of their work showed up in the spring issue of *"Search for Health"* in 1992. As soon as their critical results appeared in print, authority struck! A powerful trade organization *"The Swiss Association of Dealers in Electronic Apparatuses for Households and Industry" (FEA),* forced a Swiss Court to issue a gag order against Hertel and Blanc. That was the end of that.

I put my microwave on a skip (dumpster) shortly after the report first appeared and haven't used one since. I strongly urge you to do the same!

Life 9 – The Spiritual Cleanse

This step involves two vitally important aspects. The first stresses the supreme value of taking regular time for yourself to indulge in gentle introspection. We talked about this in *"Step 7...The Emotional Detox"*. This is a time you put aside the distractions of every-day life including smartphones and e-mails and focus on the present moment and what it brings. I urge everybody to schedule at least 10 minutes per day for this.

The second and connected issue is *"Meditation"*. Every philosophy known to man preaches the value of meditation. I have literally asked hundreds of people whether or not they meditate and invariably get the same answer.

"I can't do it!"

"It's too difficult to stop thinking."

That is precisely why it is so important. Meditation like many other healthy practices requires a little bit of discipline. It is not about sitting still and gazing into space for hours at a time like a Sadhu. All I am asking is for you to sit still for a few minutes every day. As your practice improves you will find it easy to devote more time to your meditation. The minutes will slip by un-noticed.

How to Meditate

Sit still in a comfortable position.

No need for the lotus position, sitting upright in a chair will do fine.

Hold a question in your mind. You don't have to answer the question, simply ask it.

"What am I?" is a good question.

The subconscious is programmed to come up with answers. Don't let it answer.

Then it will keep searching for more and more answers at an unconscious level.

This is a good way of silencing the ever talkative ego.

The ego's *"inner chat"* is the source of all our problems.

The purpose of meditation is to silence the talkative ego. It has been preaching negative states to you for much too long.

When you ask a question like *"What am I?"* Answers might pop up. Some of the answers could be insightful.

When an answer arrives. Ask…*"Where did that come from?"* It can only have come from you

Having understood that continue with your question mantra; *"What am I?"* and so on.

When you begin to glimpse the answer to your question…*"What am I?"* You have gone beyond the realms of the mind. You are now experiencing true meditation, and this is when the results begin to arrive. Prepare to be surprised.

Usually, the answers don't come from you, because if they did, they would prompt another round of questioning. They reach us from the world around us. They are not internal, they are external. For instance, somebody will say something that catches your attention as it provides an answer to the question you have been posing over and over again. Or you will read something in a book, a sentence or phrase will pop out in a film or on TV. Maybe somebody will post something on *"Facebook"* which will appear to hit the nail on the head. That's how it works. You need to be present and in the moment to catch the snippet. It's time we all woke up and came out of our electronically induced hypnotic trance. These realizations serve as intuitive guides to show the path you need to follow for your highest good and best intention. Slowly your life begins to change. One morning you are prompted to take a different route to work. You stop to buy a newspaper and bump into an old friend who you have not seen for years. Is this a coincidence? Jung would call it a *"synchronicity"*. He would define a *"synchronicity"* as a meaningful coincidence which has no discernible causal connection. You took a different route to work and there is no connection between that action and the meeting of your old friend. However, the meeting gave you an opportunity to re-kindle longstanding and valuable relationship that goes on to change your life in a beneficial manner.

Remember how we defined feelings to be either *"heavy"* or *"light"* in the Emotional Detox. If meeting the old friend feels light, bright and breezy to you, it is a positive situation that will more than likely take your life forward in some direction. If it is heavy the opposite might be true. However, I am certain the more time you spend in meditation, you will find overall life gets better and better. You can't ask for any more than that. I suggest you tag your meditation session onto your daily *"clearing practice"*. Start with two minutes and gradually increase the time as the meditation becomes easier. Remember to always work with a question. The ultimate question is arguably *"What am I?"* What's the answer.......Let it come, but not from you. I would hope you are an *"infinite being"*. You are aware and you have no limits. When you truly grasp the fact you are an *"infinite being"*, you have reached a high level of spiritual realization. Is this enlightenment? I don't know, but you are certainly more aware. It's a useful question too. Would an *"infinite being"* put up with such and such a situation? If the answer is *"no"*, you need to make some changes.

Nothing here in *"The Spiritual Cleanse"* involves religion. We are all Gods in our own right. Most religions tell us the opposite. Jesus was possibly the best healer the world has ever known.

Yet he explicitly tells us, we can do all he could do and perhaps even more. Why then are we not doing this? Instead, we rely on external forces, be they doctors, medicines or gurus for our healing power when it lies inside each one of us all along. Come grasp your power, use it and see the world change. The first step on that path is to touch base with yourself; the best way to make that priceless connection is to start by meditating. That is the ninth Step in *"A Cat Has Nine Lives and So Do You"*. You don't need to take my word for this. Try it yourself and see what changes in your experience. Be sure of course to always ask the right questions.

We often disempower ourselves by posing the wrong questions. A question like: *"Why can't I succeed in life?"* is a poor question. It will bring up a string of miserable answers either consciously or unconsciously. Let the subconscious run with this one and the ego will have a field day. It will search out all the reasons it can to show you why you are a failure. You will feel heavy and disempowered. Would an infinite being pose a question like that?

Instead, we need to ask a positively directed question. *"Why"* questions are preferable because they are open-ended. Open-ended questions provide terrain for open-ended answers which are empowering and make us feel light, bright and breezy. All good states, wouldn't you agree? Questions like:

"Why am I so grateful for everything I have?" Or

"Why do I allow myself to be unlimited?" These are the questions we need to be asking to enhance our state of being. Not close-ended variants requiring a simple *"yes"* or *"no"* response.

The what, why and how questioning technique provides a useful tool for overcoming problems. When a challenge rolls through the door, you need to learn to speak a new language. Here's how..... Take the negative situation and turn it into a positive question.

Instead of: *"Why do my neighbors always park so badly that it makes it difficult to reach my house?*

See that sentence is full of judgments *"park so badly"* and "*difficult to reach my house*".

Instead, let's look at this from a different angle. Have your neighbors ever blocked you from driving into your driveway? Probably not; you have been focusing on the difficulty and not the actual act of blockage. Let's change the question.

"*How is it I always been such a good driver that I have managed to get around the other cars and safely reach my driveway?*" Doesn't that feel very different? It's much lighter. It takes the sting out of the judgment and takes away the conflict. Now the situation is calm. Try this yourself. Learn to speak the new language of questions and see how it does away with tension. This might be a new approach for you. It takes you to a new place. It's so much better being "*happy*" and wrong than always being "*right*" and uptight!

One more thing before we close. Please remember the potent power of gratitude. The Medieval Cleric "Meister Eckhart" proclaimed, there is only one prayer. That is:

"*Thank you, God!*"

When we hold a thought of gratitude in mind, all negativity vanishes. Many wonderful things happen to every one of us each day of our lives. Why is it so many forget the good and focus on the bad? Why do we focus on the single event that did not work out as expected over the course of the day? Be grateful for the good and the bad will take care of itself.

Here is a powerful exercise.

The Gratitude Journal

Buy an attractive note-book

Find ten occurrences each day that you are grateful for. They don't have to be major.

Write each event into your "*Journal*". "*I am very grateful that I had delicious spinach soup for lunch.*"

Don't forget to say "*thank you*". "*I am very grateful that I had delicious spinach soup for lunch. Thank you.* "

"*I am truly grateful for the love and support showed to me by my family over the years. Thank you.*"

"*II am truly grateful for the loyalty of my clients and the trust thy have placed in me. Thank you*"

"I am truly grateful for the unconditional love given to me by my wonderful dogs. Thank you."

"I am grateful for my health which has enabled me to live happily and successfully over the years. Thank you."

Now it's your turn. Be sure to keep your *"Journal"* going for at least 30 days and notice the changes that take place in your life.

We would love feedback from you on this.

*   *   *   *   *

That brings us to the end of our *"Nine Steps"*. This is not a novel. It' a Guide Book and Manual to help you along the road to good health. Please use it wisely. We are here to help you along the road. If you require assistance to stay on track, simply send us an e-mail.

Alister Bredee

Koh Samui 2017

<u>healthambitconsultancy@protonmail.com</u>.

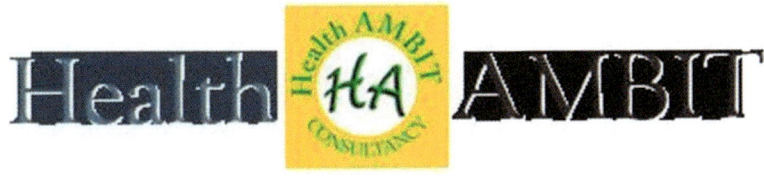

Alister Bredee

About the Author

Alister Bredee

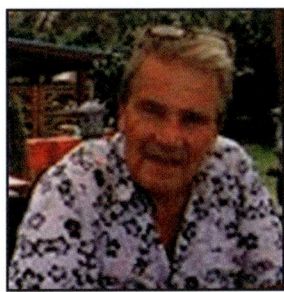

After a career spanning many years in the Middle-East, Alister Bredee decided to re-train in Psychotherapy and Hypnotherapy. He graduated in 1984 but quickly found the tools that he had learned were often cumbersome and inadequate for work with his clients. He started a long and fascinating journey to find more and better ways. This voyage took him first to Homeopathy and then to Applied Kinesiology. In 1988 he enrolled in a Holistic Medicine Programme at Howell College with a campus at London's Regent's College, beautifully situated in the midst of Regent's Park and another at Sherborne in Dorset. The Course involved residency at Sir Anton Jayasuriya;'s "Medicina Alternativa" in Colombo, Sri Lanka. He graduated as a D.HH (U.K.) M.D. (Sri Lanka) and as a Clinical Nutritionist in 1992, having established a practice in Harley Street and the prestigious Hale Clinic, again close to Regent's Park.

He moved his practice to Dublin, where he opened *"Natural Solutions"* a healing Centre beside the sea in Monkstown, South County Dublin.

Alister Bredee trained in the Meridian Energy Therapies under Dr. Tam Llewellyn and traveled to the USA to meet with Gary Craig, the founder of EFT. He became the Administrator for the Irish Association for Applied Meridian Techniques

(IAAMT). He also worked with Today's Therapist Magazine, where he taught EFT and other Meridian Energy based techniques to therapists in the UK and Ireland. He introduced his own variant which he called AMBIT (Alister's Meridian Based Integrative Therapy) which he presented at the first ACEP Conference in Europe in Switzerland and later at the second Conference at Lady Margaret Hall, part of Oxford University. He published his first book *"Full Circle"* in 2004 which outlines work with Meridian Energy Psychology

Alister moved to Thailand in 2005 and moved to Koh Samui in 2007, where he has been actively working in the *"detox"* industry ever since.

Printed in Great Britain
by Amazon